TESTIMONIALS:

"Dr. Gonzales wrote an amazing guide to tell parents when it's the right time to take their child to the orthodontists so their smile can be set straight. He is such a gifted and caring orthodontist."

—Dr. Nicole Teifer

Orthodontist

"I have known Dr. Gonzales for a number of years and this book is a reflection of the level of detail he puts into his work. He has a genuine concern for his patients. This book will help anyone who is curious about orthodontics know what to look for in a great orthodontist."

—Dr. Chase Dansie

Orthodontist

"Dr. Gonzales has truly put together a great resource for patients to learn more about the benefits of a great smile and a healthy bite. Knowing Dr. Gonzales for the past decade, I can say that he is truly one of the most relatable and humble orthodontists that I know. His office, customer service, and overall patient experience are second to none. If I weren't an orthodontist myself, I would certainly trust my children to his care."

—Dr. Jason M. Hartman

Diplomate, American Board of Orthodontics

"*Congratulations to Dr. Gonzales for a well-written and concise guide for parents considering orthodontic treatment for their children or themselves. Throughout the book, Dr. Gonzales sets things straight about orthodontics by simplifying topics that are supported by facts and references. I couldn't be prouder to state, without a doubt, that he's an amazing orthodontist, a genuinely honest person, and now a published author. Great job!*"

—Dr. David Caggiano

Orthodontist

"*The process of choosing the right orthodontist for your child or yourself can be a very daunting task when you don't know what you don't know about orthodontics. Dr. Gonzales has taken all of the guess work out of choosing an orthodontist in his new book,* Setting Them Straight. *This book will serve as a guide to help you navigate this exciting journey to acquiring your sensational new smile. Dr. Gonzales is committed to helping patients achieve the smile of their dreams and tells you how to get there from here. This is a must read for any parent or patient considering orthodontics.*"

—Dr. Kerry White Brown

Orthodontist

Setting Them
STRAIGHT

Setting Them
STRAIGHT

The Fact-Based Guide to a Spectacular Smile Through Orthodontics

DR. DANTE GONZALES

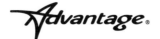

Published by Advantage, Charleston, South Carolina.
Member of Advantage Media Group.

ADVANTAGE is a registered trademark, and the Advantage colophon is a trademark of Advantage Media Group, Inc.

Printed in the United States of America.

10 9 8 7 6 5 4 3 2 1

ISBN: 978-1-59932-830-0
LCCN: 2018964304

Cover design by Carly Blake.
Layout design by Melanie Cloth.

This publication is designed to provide accurate and authoritative information in regard to the subject matter covered. It is sold with the understanding that the publisher is not engaged in rendering legal, accounting, or other professional services. If legal advice or other expert assistance is required, the services of a competent professional person should be sought.

 Advantage Media Group is proud to be a part of the Tree Neutral® program. Tree Neutral offsets the number of trees consumed in the production and printing of this book by taking proactive steps such as planting trees in direct proportion to the number of trees used to print books. To learn more about Tree Neutral, please visit **www.treeneutral.com**.

Advantage Media Group is a publisher of business, self-improvement, and professional development books and online learning. We help entrepreneurs, business leaders, and professionals share their Stories, Passion, and Knowledge to help others Learn & Grow. Do you have a manuscript or book idea that you would like us to consider for publishing? Please visit **advantagefamily.com** or call **1.866.775.1696**.

This book is dedicated to my parents, both educators, who taught me not only the value of education, but also the value of being an educator. And also to my wife, Stacey, and my children, Isabella and Marco, who fill my life with love and laughter and make my life whole. Without their unwavering support this book would never have been written.

S ince the development of the internet and the world wide web, it has become easier and easier to access to information with each year that passes. Unfortunately, much of what passes as knowledge/information on the internet is actually just opinion, anecdotes from one patient or one doctor's experience. One must always ask themselves ... Is this true? Has this been proven scientifically?

Although orthodontic devices and appliances evolve and change every decade, the principles behind orthodontic tooth movement do not. The biology of the mouth and teeth has not changed. Every year that goes by there is more and more research produced that gives us a better insight and understanding of tooth movement. The science helps us better understand how our appliances and devices work in the mouth. What Dr. Gonzales has done in this book is to help break down all of the scientific literature into understandable bite-sized pieces for the patient seeking orthodontic treatment. This book focuses on helping patients understand when to start orthodontic treatment. It also helps patients understand what is actual orthodontic science, and what is just commercial branding and hype.

The aim of this book is not to try and review every single type of orthodontic treatment (that would take several volumes of books), it does cover many of the principles behind orthodontics. It also helps patients understand what goes into diagnosing and treatment planning an orthodontic case. Many patients and parents think that by just going to their dentist everything should turn out okay. However, many dental problems have a solution in orthodontic treatment. However, many dentists lack the training and knowledge to understand how to deal with these problems. They may even go unnoticed by the dentist. This book tries to explain what many of those problems are and why it's important for a child to visit an orthodontist at the appropriate age. More importantly, it explains why it is important to not wait for a dentist referral. Many dentists cannot or do not recognize many of these problems until it is very late, or sometimes too late to treat. A dentist's main focus is on cavities and periodontal disease. In many dentist offices there is very little attention paid to the growth and development of a patient's proper skeletal or dental development.

One of the biggest frustrations that many orthodontists face, including myself, is that patients that are seeking orthodontic treatment get many differing opinions and ideas on what should be done to them or their child. Parents and patients are getting their information on the internet, or worse, going to several orthodontic consultations and then choosing the treatment option they hear the most. For example, if three orthodontists say their case cannot be treated with Invisalign, and the fourth says that it can, that doesn't mean that the case cannot be treated with Invisalign. The reality is that maybe three of the four orthodontists are not experienced enough with using Invisalign to treat that case. Patients are weighing the opinions of all the orthodontists and then choosing the majority of those opinions. While this may be better than choosing the first orthodontist you see. It would be much wiser to get information from an orthodontist that practices evidence-based treatment and has no financial interest in your child's treatment.

Dr. Dustin Burleson

Making a Difference

decided to become an orthodontist because I learned, firsthand, the ability orthodontics has to make a positive difference in someone's life. What I found, however, was that dental schools did little to address orthodontics and what education there was on the specialty was very sparse. It was almost like a secret society.

It wasn't until I became an orthodontic resident that I was finally able to learn the complexities and principles of this specialized field. After I'd read several hundred orthodontic journal articles, I began to appreciate the science and principles behind it.

I've had a private practice for over twenty years, and I've seen many patients who should have been referred to my office years before they came in because their dentist had little—if any—orthodontic education. Because of this lack of training, those dentists often misunderstood their patients' orthodontic needs or they believed

1

orthodontics wasn't necessary; for instance, if the patient still had deciduous (baby) teeth present. Just because baby teeth are present doesn't mean a patient can't benefit from orthodontic treatment. In fact, the ideal age for a first orthodontic exam is seven years old, when children are still losing their first baby teeth and may not have lost any yet. An exam at this age can catch problems as they first start to develop, and can make a huge difference in patients' future.

However, if dentists know little about orthodontics, the general public would know even less. In fact, I often find myself fielding questions about orthodontics stemming from false statements on the internet or correcting rumors about long-standing myths and fad treatments.

The ignorance and proliferation of false information regarding orthodontics is what brought me to write this book. Even though the internet is full of dental and orthodontic information, it's difficult for many patients to know what information is based in science and what isn't.

I want to help patients and the parents of young patients understand the principles of orthodontics, and what is possible with orthodontic treatment and what is not. While orthodontics can make incredible changes with a patient's smile and their bite, it's not magic; we're still bound by the principles and biology of the mouth. For example, a certain procedure may be possible for one patient, but it may not be possible—or have the same effect—on a different patient due to their differing anatomies. I've seen many patients who would have benefited from knowing many of these principles before undergoing treatment, or before electing to receive treatment that ended up being unnecessary. Other patients could have received more timely treatment and avoided tooth extraction or orthodontic surgery if they'd known to visit an orthodontist earlier on.

If you're interested in the facts of a specific orthodontic principle, this book is designed so that you can flip to that section and learn the answer. However, I invite you to read the book fully and learn about the evolution of orthodontics.

This book will help patients by answering common questions concerning orthodontics, explaining many of its principles, and describing what is and is not possible with orthodontics. I hope it arms you with the information you need to make better-informed decisions and that it helps you achieve the smile of your dreams.

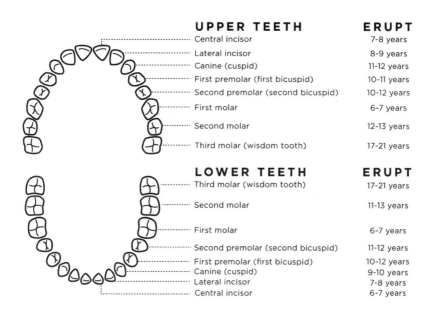

UPPER TEETH	**ERUPT**
Central incisor	7-8 years
Lateral incisor	8-9 years
Canine (cuspid)	11-12 years
First premolar (first bicuspid)	10-11 years
Second premolar (second bicuspid)	10-12 years
First molar	6-7 years
Second molar	12-13 years
Third molar (wisdom tooth)	17-21 years

LOWER TEETH	**ERUPT**
Third molar (wisdom tooth)	17-21 years
Second molar	11-13 years
First molar	6-7 years
Second premolar (second bicuspid)	11-12 years
First premolar (first bicuspid)	10-12 years
Canine (cuspid)	9-10 years
Lateral incisor	7-8 years
Central incisor	6-7 years

CHAPTER 1

How Are Orthodontists and Dentists Different?

What is an orthodontist? Better yet, why are there orthodontists in the first place? To answer the first question, an orthodontist is a specialist in dentistry who completes an extra two to three years of education to learn how to correctly align teeth and jaws, as well as how to diagnose, treat, and prevent dental and facial irregularities.[1]

But to answer the second question, we need to step back in time.

Humans have been interested in straightening their teeth since ancient Egyptian times. Mummified Egyptians have been found with gold bands wrapped around their teeth, which researchers believed

---

1   "What We Do," American Association of Orthodontists, accessed September 2017, https://www.aaoinfo.org/about/what-we-do.

were laced with catgut in an attempt to either close space between teeth or prevent unwanted shifting.[2]

But the Egyptians weren't alone in their efforts. Many other ancient cultures found ways to manipulate teeth in order to improve their appearance or to correct a bad bite, also known as a *malocclusion*. Between 500 and 300 BC, both Hippocrates and Aristotle spoke of diseases of the teeth and various treatment methods, from extraction to the use of wires to hold loose teeth or broken jaws in place. By AD 166, the Etruscans had developed dental prosthetics that we may consider modern, such as fixed bridgework and gold crowns,[3] and in the early eighteenth century, French dentist Pierre Fauchard used a u-shaped piece of iron called a *blandeau* to expand arches.[4]

Modern orthodontics, however, didn't begin to appear until the 1800s, when the invention of vulcanized rubber spurred dental inventors to come up with new appliances to improve the alignment of the teeth and bite.

EARLY INNOVATIONS IN ORTHODONTIC APPLIANCES

- **1819**—Christophe-Francois Delabarre invents the "wire crib," a half-moon–shaped device attached directly to the tooth to help straighten it.

---

2   "Braces, Pointless and Essential," *The Atlantic*, accessed September 2017, https://www.theatlantic.com/health/archive/2015/07/braces-dentures-history/397934/.

3   "History of Dentistry Timeline," American Dental Association, accessed September 2017, http://www.ada.org/en/about-the-ada/ada-history-and-presidents-of-the-ada/ada-history-of-dentistry-timeline.

4   "The History of Dental Braces," Dr. Jaw Orthodontists, accessed September 2017, http:// /blog/history-dental-braces/.

- **1843**—Edward Maynard first uses gum elastics attached to wire to align the jaw.

- **1850**—E. J. Tucker uses rubber bands cut from rubber tubing instead of wire to help align the jaw.

- **1893**—Henry A. Baker uses Delabarre's wire crib and Tucker's rubber bands to create an improved jaw alignment system.

- **1899**—Dr. Edward Angle invents the modern orthodontic appliance: metal bands tensioned with wire to straighten teeth.

- **1900–Present Day**—Orthodontists and engineers have designed better, more efficient brackets and orthodontic appliances. They are all modifications on Dr. Angle's original appliance using bands and wires.

THE LAUNCH OF MODERN ORTHODONTICS

The beginning of modern orthodontics can be traced back to 1900, when Dr. Edward Angle founded of the Angle School of Orthodontia in St. Louis, Missouri.[5] This was the first time orthodontics was formalized as a dental specialty. Before then, most dentists dabbled in some orthodontics, but no one solely focused their practice in that one specialty.

---

5 "History of Dentistry Timeline," American Dental Association, accessed September 2017, http://www.ada.org/en/about-the-ada/ada-history-and-presidents-of-the-ada/ada-history-of-dentistry-timeline.

At Dr. Angle's school, dentists were able to take a post-graduate course on how to straighten teeth using appliances that Angle himself had developed. These appliances were some of the first to be directly affixed to the teeth using materials such as steel and sometimes gold.

Thanks to Dr. Angle, orthodontics is considered the first and oldest specialty in dentistry, and Angle is revered as the founding father of modern orthodontics.

From 1900 on, dentists who wanted to perform orthodontics would go to a post-graduate orthodontic school for additional education in this specialty—a tradition that continues to this day.

Becoming an orthodontist isn't easy, however. Dentists looking to pursue this specialty must apply to an orthodontic residency after graduating dental school and be accepted to the program, which are highly sought after by dental students. Due to the competitiveness, orthodontic programs tend to only take dental students who are at or near the top of their class and have great scores on their national board exams. Average doesn't fly in orthodontics.

For instance, when I graduated from dental school, I was at the top of my class of 150 students and had received a ninety-ninth percentile score on my national board exam. And yet, of the ten programs I applied for, I was only accepted by three.

Most orthodontic programs have anywhere from 300 to 600 applicants vying for two to ten resident positions. In my case, the program I chose to attend had 540 applicants for four positions. It's not an easy specialty to get into, and when you do, it's a challenging and rigorous program to complete.

THE ORTHODONTIST IN TRAINING

Most orthodontic programs range in length from twenty-four to thirty-six months and involve 6,000 to 8,000 hours of training and studying. During that time, the resident learns how to diagnose everything that can negatively affect the teeth, the alignment of the teeth, facial deformities, and the bite—from skeletal discrepancies between the upper and lower jaws to skeletal discrepancies between the jaw and the skull. They learn how the jaw develops and how the teeth develop and erupt in the mouth. They learn what causes the crowding and misalignment of teeth, and they learn multiple different techniques and strategies to address these problems and even correct them before they occur, if the patient gets to them early enough.

Sometimes, just by taking out a baby tooth at the right time, for instance, you can avoid a lot of problems down the road. Or, by placing fixed or removable appliances on permanent teeth, an orthodontist can treat discrepancies before they become so aberrant that only jaw surgery can correct them.

From treating obvious issues to mending problems unapparent to the untrained eye, orthodontics goes well beyond the training of a typical four-year dental program. In most dental schools, orthodontics tends to be treated as a tertiary topic, glossed over in favor of the main dental procedures of fillings, crowns, bridges, root canals, tooth extractions, and learning how to treat periodontal diseases and gingivitis.

I recall only spending about twenty to thirty hours of the entire four years of dental school on orthodontics. Most of the orthodontic education centered on very simple things like recognizing what an over or underbite looks like and knowing that you need to call an orthodontist when you see those conditions. It wasn't that we weren't willing to study these conditions, but there's simply not enough time to learn both general dentistry and orthodontics at the same time.

Orthodontics already intrigued me, and I was fortunate to match with a great orthodontics resident during our dental school's ten-week rotation through the orthodontics department. He helped me treat a case during my time there—a case that will always stand out to me because of how excited the patient was with the results.

It was a short and simple case, wherein we basically moved one of the patient's front teeth out of a crossbite and back into alignment with the adjacent teeth using a removable, retainer-like appliance. It was a condition that the forty-five-year-old patient had lived with her whole life. When she saw it corrected, she practically went through the roof with excitement, and right then and there I knew that I was hooked on becoming an orthodontist.

SPECIALIZING IN A WORLD OF RAPIDLY ADVANCING TECHNOLOGY

For all dental professionals, education doesn't end at graduation. In most states, there is a yearly minimum of twenty-five hours of continued education required, which is important due to the rapid advancement of new techniques created, mostly by the increasing number of new digital tools and new dental materials available.

Keeping up with all of the advancements and what you need to know in your own particular field of dentistry leaves little room to learn other specialties, such as pediatric dentistry, oral surgery, or orthodontics, to a level of competency. For instance, in order to just keep up with everything that's going on in orthodontics, I end up enrolling in anywhere from twenty-five to fifty hours of continued education every year.

With this incredible growth in mind, one must ask: How can a dentist be good at orthodontics and yet still be a good dentist?

DENTISTS THAT "DO" ORTHODONTICS

There's a dirty little secret about dentistry: the field is overproducing dentists. According to a 2014 study conducted by the American Dental Association's Health Policy Institute, "The per capita supply of dentists in the United States is projected to increase through 2033. Total inflows to the dentist workforce are expected to exceed total outflows, and the net gain is expected to exceed the growth in the U.S. population." That is, we'll have more dentists graduating college by 2033 than we'll have dentists retiring—at a rate that will exceed our total population growth.[6]

With so much competition in dentistry, the typical dentist must find ways to stand out. Unfortunately, this often means expanding their repertoire of procedures into areas in which they have little formal training.

For instance, dentists may offer not only cleanings, fillings, and cavity restoration, but also periodontal procedures, orthodontics, and oral surgery—all areas that dentists used to refer out to specialists but are now being offered in-house to boost office revenue. Instead of two to three years of training in these specialties, however, these dentists are relying on the training they received in three-day weekend courses or courses offered over several weekends.

Many of these courses cover the basics of orthodontic diagnosis and treatment, such as how to diagnose a bad bite (malocclusion), how to put on braces, which wires to use, and how to straighten out

---

6   Bradly Munson and Marko Vujicic, "Supply of Dentists in the United States is Likely to Grow," *American Dental Association*, October 2014, http://www.ada. org/~/media/ADA/Science%20and%20Research/HPI/Files/HPIBrief_1014_1.ashx.

the "smile" teeth (the first six visible teeth in your mouth). There is very little on how to finish a case with a proper, functional bite.

These courses, however, don't focus on the vital interrelationships of bite, jaw, and tooth position in relation to facial aesthetics. Instead, they only touch on the basics, which means dentists who attend these weekend orthodontic courses do not gain a full understanding of what their patients need and how to really fix it.

For example, during a typical orthodontic residency program, a resident may spend a whole year taking a course in cephalometrics, which is the study of the head x-rays taken by most orthodontists. If these weekend courses touch on cephalometrics at all, it's maybe a few hours at most.

Dentists leave these weekend programs with cursory knowledge of the subject or procedures. They're not learning how to diagnose a case properly, and their patients will not get the best treatment options, because without the best diagnosis, you're not going to get the best treatment. If your dentist can't understand the core of your problem, how is he or she going to fix it?

TREATING THE CAUSE, NOT THE EFFECT

One of the most common problems I see when dental colleagues attempt orthodontic treatments is not understanding the core issues that created the problem in the first place, like crooked teeth or a bad bite. More-knowledgeable dentists have a bit more expertise and ability to diagnose what the problem may be but may not be versed in the treatment plan needed to correct the problem.

For example, dentists often fail to see skeletal discrepancies, tooth size discrepancies, or a number of other issues that may not be visible to the untrained eye. Or they believe that you don't need to take out teeth to correct overcrowding; they think that all you need to do is expand the jaw. Expanding the upper jaw may alleviate the need for extractions in a very small percentage of cases, but in the vast majority of cases, this may also be contraindicated—meaning that trying to expand the jaws will create more problems than it will solve.

Many dentists fail to realize that the lower jaw cannot be expanded—it's a single, solid bone. You can shift the teeth away from the tongue and expand the arch, but that's rarely advisable. When the teeth are moved outward for alignment, they are being moved into the outer portion of the bony support structure. The upper jaw can be expanded, because it's made of two separate plates, but again, the overall harmony of the jaw relationship must be kept in mind. If widened too much, the upper jaw could be expanded beyond the lower jaw and create a bite that is not coordinated—a bite that can be awkward and uncomfortable.

In one particular case, I remember seeing a patient whose dentist, in order to avoid extractions, had expanded her upper jaw so far out that her upper teeth didn't come in proper contact with her lower teeth, and her lower teeth were expanded so far out that they were at the edge of their support structures. The patient's bone and gums were so thin that she was likely going to have a lot recession in those areas in the next several years.

There was little I could do for her at that point except recommend moving her teeth back to their ideal position, which likely meant taking out some teeth to prevent the crowding that she was trying to correct in the first place.

Many patients have come to me over the years with the same complaint resulting from dentist-conducted orthodontic procedures: either their teeth aren't as straight as they want them to be, or their bite just doesn't feel right—or both. On the other hand, the case treated by the orthodontist usually will have a better finish, a more ideal bite, and a more aesthetic result. There are dentists out there who can produce good orthodontic work, but it is usually after years or decades of practice. When comparing the results of cases, most cases finished by orthodontists will have a more ideal result versus cases finished by dentists.

Not too long ago, a dentist asked for my help following a braces procedure he conducted. He was trying to straighten out his patient's teeth but couldn't figure out why there was such a large overjet created between the upper and lower teeth after they were aligned ("overbite" refers to the overlapping of the upper teeth over the lower teeth, while "overjet" describes when the upper teeth stick out significantly beyond the lower teeth). I noticed that the patient had a large Class 2 molar relationship—that is, there was a large discrepancy between the upper and lower teeth because of the bite. The lower jaw was too far back to meet the upper jaw with the teeth in an ideal bite. The dentist didn't realize this, and by straightening the patient's teeth, he also created an overjet of about eight millimeters.

In another case presented to me about five or six years ago, a twenty-eight-year-old woman routinely saw a dentist to close down an anterior open bite, which is where the front teeth don't meet and jut out as though the tongue has been pressing against them (which it often has). In trying to push those teeth back in, the dentist had pulled down the woman's upper teeth so much so that when she smiled, she showed almost three-quarters of an inch of gums.

When she came to me, she broke down crying, saying that her dentist had made her look like a horse and begged me to fix it. When I told her that the only way to fix her condition at that point was a type of jaw/face operation called orthognathic surgery, she almost became hysterical.

She had trusted her dentist to know what he was doing with the procedures, and also it costed less than going to an orthodontist. In the end, if she were to undergo the orthognathic surgery, it would've cost her anywhere from $18,000 to $25,000.

This was all because her dentist failed to really look at her facial structure, conduct a cephalometric analysis (basically an x-ray and analysis of the head), and account for skeletal issues. The dentist didn't realize the young woman's out-thrust teeth weren't due to the position of her teeth, but rather the position of her jaws and how they diverged from each other. Any orthodontist conducting a simple cephalometric analysis would've seen this and treated her in a way that altered the skeletal relationship to repair the cause—such as with temporary anchorage devices or by going directly into surgery—instead of spending years in costly braces first.

But the dentist, only seeing the out-thrust teeth, chose to treat the effect and not the cause. And the end result was far from ideal.

COMMON PATIENT RESULTS CAUSED BY MINIMAL ORTHODONTIC TRAINING

- bite feels "off"
- patient doesn't like the final appearance of teeth
- teeth not aligned correctly
- teeth pushed out too far
- overcrowding issues are not addressed properly (tooth mass not reduced)

Most of the problems dentists make center around the bite, because the easiest procedure in orthodontics is to put braces on or to put an Invisalign tray in someone's mouth. On the other hand, one of the hardest things to do in orthodontics is achieve an ideal finish, where all the teeth fit together properly and are in harmony with the surrounding bone and facial structures.

Finishing a case to the ideal is where orthodontists thrive, but for dentists, the focus is less on the bite and more in straightening the teeth. They just don't have the knowledge and techniques to correct the bite.

Practicing orthodontics in a dental office isn't illegal, of course, just like it's not illegal for an oral surgeon to perform nose surgery or do a breast augmentation. But most people would say it's not recommended and that you should probably see a specialist for these procedures.

So, the question is, who do you want doing your orthodontics?

COMMON QUESTIONS: DENTIST VERSUS ORTHODONTIST

Q: Are my teeth going to be any straighter if I see an orthodontist instead of a dentist?

A: A lot of the time what patients really mean by this question is, "Straight teeth are straight teeth are straight teeth. Why does it matter who straightens my teeth as long as they're straight?"

The thing is, there's more to orthodontics than just straightening teeth, and straightening teeth isn't as easy as putting on braces or using an Invisalign tray. Once you start moving teeth, all kinds of things can happen. The key is in knowing how to avert these problems before they occur and, if they do occur, knowing how to fix them.

Q: Why does an orthodontist's treatment cost so much more than what my dentist is charging?

A: The difference is due to the experience and training that an orthodontist has over a dentist, as well as the orthodontist's ability to finish a case. Anyone can put braces or Invisalign in your mouth and start the process, but finishing the case is where all 7,000 hours of training plus hundreds of hours of continuing education come into play: in finishing that orthodontic case to the ideal.

Chapter 1 Summary

- Orthodontics is a specialization of dentistry that involves an additional two to three years of training and education on how to correctly align teeth and jaws, as well as how to diagnose, treat, and prevent dental and facial irregularities.

- Humans have been attempting to straighten teeth since the days of ancient Egypt.

- Modern orthodontics can officially be traced back to the opening of the Angle School of Orthodontia in St. Louis, Missouri in 1900. Dr. Edward Angle is considered the founding father of modern orthodontics.

- Orthodontic programs are notoriously difficult to get into and typically only take dental students who graduated top of their class and have very high scores on their national board exams.

- Most orthodontic programs range in length from twenty-four to thirty-six months and involve 6,000 to 8,000 hours of training.

- Dental schools rarely spend much time on learning dental specialties such as orthodontics, oral surgery, and endodontics.

- Orthodontists focus on learning how the jaw develops, how the teeth develop and erupt in the mouth, and what causes the crowding and misalignment of teeth. They learn different techniques and strategies to address these problems and even prevent them before they occur.

- To stand out in the dental field, more dentists are offering procedures that are typically referred out to specialists.

- To train for these specialized procedures, dentists will often take weekend courses that only focus on the basic procedure and not on the bigger picture of what may be causing the issue to begin with (i.e., they may not be able to provide a proper diagnosis).

- Dentists may start procedures such as braces but may not have the knowledge and training to properly finish these cases. This is where orthodontists excel—finishing to the ideal.

The Benefits and Realities of Orthodontics

The majority of people who walk into an orthodontic practice are looking to improve their smile. It's usually their highest priority, whether it has to do with an overbite, underbite, crowding, or just crooked teeth. Their main goal is to improve the teeth that show in their smile. When a patient needs to undergo a complex and lengthy orthodontic treatment, they will often ask, "Can't you just straighten my front teeth in six or seven months?" What most patients don't realize is that in some cases, just straightening out the front teeth may actually take their bite from bad to worse.

A smaller number of patients will come to us for bite issues. They may feel like their bite is off or that it's not functioning correctly—something we call a *functioning occlusion*—but the vast majority are concerned first and foremost with straightening their teeth.

However, correcting their bite, or *occlusion*, is often far more complex than just slapping on some braces and walking out six months later with the perfect smile.

MORE THAN "JUST STRAIGHTENING TEETH"

Of course, there are occasional patients who come in to get their teeth straightened and don't care whether or not their bite is functioning properly and in harmony with the rest of their mouth. As orthodontists, we would be doing those patients a disservice by leaving them with a bad bite. Doing so could lead to numerous problems down the road, including the worsening of issues they might already be suffering from, which includes, but is not limited to:

- chipping
- fracturing
- tooth loss
- excessive wear
- poor chewing ability
- problems with the jaw joint

So, when we tell patients what we'll need to do to straighten their teeth, they are often surprised at the number of steps needed. Our response is that straightening teeth is complex. We have to go through these steps to make sure we're not just improving how their teeth look, but also how the teeth fit together and function overall.

We also need to correct other aspects of their bite that will benefit the patient for a lifetime.

In a way, it's a lot like losing weight. Patients may want to lose weight to look better and feel better about themselves immediately, but doctors want the patients to lose weight to benefit their long-term health. For instance, every pound that people move away from their ideal healthy weight makes their bodies unhealthier, just as every degree that a person's teeth move away from an ideal bite leaves their mouth and body that much unhealthier.

At the same time, losing weight isn't just about lowering the number on the scale; it's about doing so in a healthy manner that doesn't deteriorate the patient's health. Instead, it improves it, and the same goes for orthodontics.

When patients come in looking to improve their smiles for their own self-esteem or just to look better, they should realize not only do their orthodontists want the same for them, but they also want their patients to have a better bite and improved function of their teeth so that their teeth can last longer and be healthier. Ultimately, that's the goal of any orthodontist.

BENEFITS OF A PROPER BITE

An ideal, functional bite—that is, when only certain teeth touch as the jaw moves around—both allows the mouth to function at optimal levels and also helps prevent issues like excessive wear and tear on the jaw joint. In an ideal bite, teeth fit together the way nature intended them to fit together. In an ideal, functional bite, there are contacts made between certain teeth. And depending on the chewing movement, the teeth are meant to function a specific way, and there are certain teeth that should hit first. For instance, when a patient slides their lower jaw forward into an edge-to-edge incisor position, none of the back teeth should be touching. The contacts during movement are called *protective excursions* and help the teeth function properly, which in turn help the teeth last longer. In addition, because the teeth are being moved to the middle of their support structures (such as the jaw bone and gums), they are in a much healthier position, with maximum support.

Additionally, improvements in the bite can help protect against general injuries and trauma, such as wear and tear from parafunctional habits such as teeth clenching and grinding, as well as prevent injuries from traumas such as sports injuries or falls. A patient with a deep overbite may suffer from excessive wear on the lower front teeth, however, if a patient has a deep overbite and grinds their teeth at night, the problem is compounded.

Then there's the overall benefit to mouth health and cleanliness. When the teeth are aligned properly, the natural cleansing mechanisms from the saliva and tongue are more effective, and the aesthetic appearance of a properly aligned bite is often a source of pride. Patients who like their smile and feel good about how their teeth are positioned in their mouths also tend to have more self-confidence and are more diligent about taking care of their teeth.

Finally, there's the benefit of improved skeletal relationships between the upper and lower jaws, which not only ensures a healthier jaw joint, but can also help with chewing, speech, and a more balanced, improved profile. When it comes to chewing, for instance, a bad bite can make it difficult to eat certain foods. In one case, I had a patient who had basically been functioning off of only two teeth in the back of her mouth. None of her other teeth touched, which made it difficult for her to eat anything solid. For years, her poor bite determined what she could eat, and in turn, her diet and nutrition suffered. Once we were able to achieve an ideal bite for her, fresh fruit, vegetables, and salads became more prominent in her diet. Her overall health improved, and she lost about thirty pounds that first year.

Speech, too, can be affected by an improper bite. While a lot of speech is muscular in nature, the structure of the mouth around the lips, tongue, and palate, as well as the influence of the teeth and bones, can play a big role in our ability to speak clearly.

BITE COMPLICATIONS THAT CAN AFFECT SPEECH

- **Crossbite**: When the overlap of the upper jaw over lower, or vice versa, is extreme (such as with overbites and underbites), the ability to pronounce letters such as s, z, and l can be compromised, forcing these letters to be pronounced with a t, n, or d sound.

- **Open bite**: When either the upper or lower jaw is forced outward so far that the teeth don't touch those on the other jaw, the same pronunciation problems found with a crossbite can occur. However, with an open bite, the ability to pronounce s sounds can be particularly challenging.

- **Overjet**: If the space between the upper and lower front teeth is greater than an average of about two mm—resulting in what's commonly called "buck teeth," where the upper jaw sticking out further than the lower—then the result can be an audible "hissing" effect with sibilant sounds such as *s* and *z*.

While the sounds are not created by the teeth, the lips and tongue use the teeth to create many of the sibilant sounds (*s, z, sh, zh, ch,* and *j*). Abnormalities of the front teeth can interfere with the tongue tip and the lips. Sometimes the tongue can adapt to these abnormalities, but the sounds still may not sound ideal. Moreover, a narrow maxillary (upper) arch can cause distorted speech and resonance because it limits the amount of space for the tongue to move within the mouth.

There are numerous reasons why having an ideal bite is the best thing for mouth health and health overall, but in general, teeth that are in the ideal position are not as likely to have complications (such as gum and bone disease, gingivitis, and periodontal disease), are more adept at clear speech, and are more resistant to injury and trauma.

THE IMPORTANCE OF A BEAUTIFUL SMILE

The visual appeal of having a straight and healthy smile can be a life-changing experience. Orthodontics can take shy, embarrassed children and give them the confidence to engage and participate in every aspect of their life. According to a perception study conducted by research firm Kelton in 2012, "Nearly three in four (73%) Americans would be more likely to trust someone with a nice smile than someone with a good job, outfit, or car," and "87% would forego something for a year in order to have a nice smile for the rest of their life," among other findings.[7] Another study has shown that 80 percent of respondents noticed someone's smile before anything else.

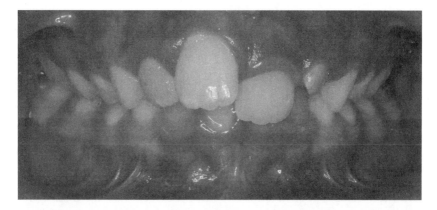

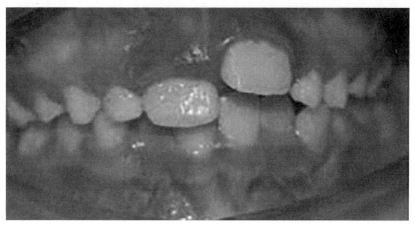

In our orthodontic practice in Dublin, California, we treat several kids a year just because of these psychosocial factors. In the age of social media and smartphones, children especially are increasingly self-conscious about their image. They're often embarrassed about their teeth, either because they're being teased at school or because it

---

7   Invisalign, "First Impressions Are Everything: New Study Confirms People With Straight Teeth Are Perceived as More Successful, Smarter and Having More Dates," PR Newswire, April 19, 2012, http://www.prnewswire.com/news-releases/first-impressions-are-everything-new-study-confirms-people-with-straight-teeth-are-perceived-as-more-successful-smarter-and-having-more-dates-148073735.html.

bothers them personally. We even have some kids as young as eight or nine asking their parents for braces to get rid of gaps or overbites. It's surprising sometimes how aware kids are of their teeth, and it's rewarding to treat them, too. Their excitement when they finally remove their braces and share their perfect smiles with the world is palpable, and their confidence is contagious.

Adults will often come to our practice to have their teeth straightened, because they feel a straighter smile will help with their job or work environment. For example, if they're hoping for a promotion to an executive position, applying for a new job, or just have to speak with people on a regular basis, they want to get their teeth straightened to improve their overall appearance.

Their concern is a real one. The condition of a smile can potentially affect a person's job prospects. A study published in 2014 by the American Association of Orthodontists found that "Persons with ideal smiles are considered more intelligent and have a greater chance of finding a job when compared with persons with nonideal smiles."[8]

What was particularly interesting about this study was that it wasn't based on hiring managers' opinions of job candidates with good teeth versus different candidates who have bad teeth. Instead, it involved showing one group of participants the original photo of a person smiling and showing their real, crooked teeth, and showing a second group of managers an image of the same person with their bite digitally corrected to appear straight. What the researchers discovered was that the candidate images with the digitally corrected smiles were consistently given higher scores by the participating hiring managers, evaluating the altered images "as superior with

---

8   MM Pithon et al., "Do dental esthetics have any influence on finding a job?" *Am J Orthod Dento facial Orthop* 146, no.4 (October 2014): 423–9, doi:10.1016/j. ajodo.2014.07.001.

respect to intelligence" compared to "the same subjects with nonideal dental esthetics."

Whether or not it's right for people to form opinions about others based on their smile, the fact is that we all, on some level, judge others by their aesthetics—at least initially. So, when it comes to self-esteem and self-confidence, straightening teeth can have a huge impact on kids and adults alike.

BETTER BITE FOR BETTER BREATHING

Another area of oral health orthodontists are in a prime position to help with, especially in adolescents, is the condition of sleep apnea, or sleep-disordered breathing. The orthodontist may not be the first type of doctor that people think to ask about sleep apnea or better breathing, but orthodontists are some of the best doctors to see for opening up a constricted airway.

Many times, the issue of an airway narrowing or closing during sleep is directly due to the shape of the palate and the position of the tongue. What orthodontists can do is widen the palate, either with certain types of expansion appliances for children or through surgery with adults.

Orthodontists can also advance the lower jaw, bringing it more in harmony with the upper jaw and allowing the airway to open up. By bringing the lower jaw forward, the tongue moves forward too, and away from the back of the throat. This causes the airway to open more.

Even if a patient is treated for sleep-disordered breathing with a separate surgical procedure, such as a tonsillectomy or adenoidectomy, the removal of those lymph nodes may not be enough to open up the airway. Sometimes you need to do skeletal changes as well, adjusting the jaw and palate to move the tongue forward and away from the back of the throat.

SLEEP APNEA/SLEEP-DISORDERED BREATHING AND ADHD

According to the National Sleep Foundation, attention-deficit/hyperactivity disorder (ADHD) "is linked with a variety of sleep problems," including sleep-disordered breathing.[9] The article went on to quote from a study published in the *Journal of Sleep Research*, which "found that treating sleep problems may be enough to eliminate attention and hyperactivity issues for some children."[10]

The article also brought up the potential link between sleep problems and ADHD in adults, quoting an additional study in which "researchers compared adults with narcolepsy, idiopathic hypersomnia, and ADHD and found a high percentage of symptom overlap, suggesting the possibility of ADHD misdiagnosis among adults."[11]

Children and adults alike who have been diagnosed with ADHD should seriously consider seeing an ear, nose, and throat (ENT) doctor, as well as having a sleep study and an orthodontic evaluation done. Over the years, I've known several patients with ADHD and behavioral issues who were evaluated for sleep apnea and treated orthodontically. In turn, their ADHD or behavioral issues just disappeared.

---

9   "ADHD and Sleep," National Sleep Foundation, accessed September 2017, https://sleepfoundation.org/sleep-disorders-problems/adhd-and-sleep.

10   S. Shur-Fen Gau, "Prevalence of sleep problems and their association with inattention/hyperactivity among children aged 6-15 in Taiwan," *J Sleep Res* 15, no. 4 (December 2006): 403–1, doi:10.1111/j.1365-2869.2006.00552.x.

11   M. Osterloo et al., "Possible confusion between primary hypersomnia and adult attention-deficit/hyperactivity disorder," *Psychiatry Res* 143, no.2-3 (August 30, 2006): 293–7, doi:10.1016/j.psychres.2006.02.009.

This whole area of sleep apnea and ADHD is still relatively new, and there are many studies being done to discover the link between sleep and ADHD. However, there are more and more cases every year that show orthodontic treatment creating improvement in sleep and, consequently, improvement in the patient's ADHD.

MAIN CAUSES OF SLEEP APNEA

There are two main causes of sleep apnea:

1.   A complication with the central nervous system (CNS).

2.   A structural obstruction, such as enlarged tonsils.

CNS-oriented sleep apnea is rare and is typically caused by a brain disorder that doesn't allow the patient to sleep well. Instead, the vast majority of patients with sleep apnea have some type of structural obstruction, usually from soft tissues such as the adenoid (the large tonsil at the back of the nasal cavity), the tonsils, or the nasal turbinates (tonsil-like ridges of tissue that line the inside of the nose). If any of these soft tissues become enlarged or constricted, they can block airways and make breathing difficult. The tongue can also cause hindered breathing if it becomes enlarged and/or falls to the back of the throat during sleep.

Allergies can play a significant role in sleep issues. Allergies can cause inflammation, especially if those soft tissues block airways, forcing breaths through the mouth and possibly contributing to difficulty sleeping. For children, especially very young children, regular allergies that result in mouth-breathing can have a negative effect on their palate development.

If children can breathe through their nose, for instance, then their mouth is closed and their tongue naturally presses against their palate, helping to shape it as it develops. If the mouth is open, however, whether from allergies or anything else, the jaw will naturally sit further back during sleep, which may prevent the palate from expanding. At the same time, the developing soft tissue, such as the tonsils and adenoid, will be more inclined to follow gravity and grow down and back, potentially reducing the size of the airway. Then, if the tongue follows and starts to sit more in the back of the throat, the airway can become even more constricted.

Being overweight can also contribute to these problems, as the additional mass can enlarge the soft tissues and make the situation worse. A person who might only have mild sleep apnea but is overweight may develop moderate sleep apnea because of it, though you don't need to be overweight to have sleep apnea.

In most cases, however, if a CNS issue isn't causing the sleep apnea, then improving the width of the palate can treat the condition. This not only helps open up the back of the throat but also gives the tongue more space. At the same time, advancing the lower jaw can also open up that space and improve breathing.

CREATING FACIAL BALANCE

Orthodontics can also do a lot to improve facial balance. For example, lip competence—your ability to close your lips together just by closing your mouth—and lip profile can both benefit from orthodontic treatment.

Reducing the angle at which the front teeth stick out can often treat lip competence and profile issues, particularly in patients suffering from a condition called *bimaxillary protrusion*, or the tendency of both jaws to jut out in a way that makes the lower half of the face look like it's pressing outward.

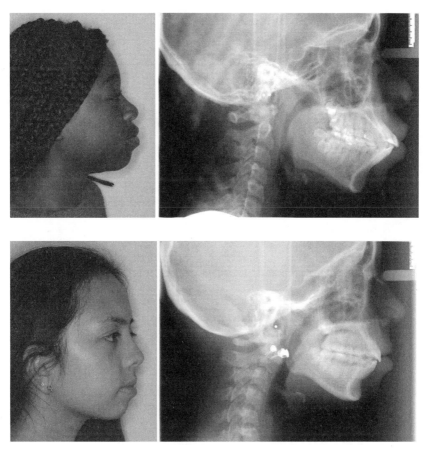

*Patients exhibiting bimaxillary protrusion and lip strain. Notice the
flexing of the muscles around the chin in order to close the lips.*

With bimaxillary protrusion, patients often have to forcefully flex
their lip muscles together to close them. Over time, this can cause
their muscles to produce a kind of dimpled-chin look, also known
as the "golf ball effect." By moving the teeth together into better
alignment with the skeletal structure, the lips and soft tissue structures can return to their ideal positions, resulting in better lip competence and profile.

Patients with the opposite condition, where the teeth lean too
far back into the mouth, can also benefit from bringing the teeth

into proper alignment and giving them a little more projection and support.

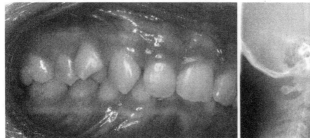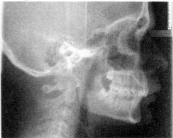

Notice how the front teeth are tipped inward and creating a deep overbite.

Additionally, there are patients who come in with narrow arches; one of their chief complaints is that others can see a lot of their teeth when they smile. In a lot of these cases, what orthodontists can do is widen the arch in a way that keeps the smile harmonious with the lips and soft tissues while also allowing the teeth to fill in the smile comfortably, ultimately giving the patient a wider and more pleasing smile.

There are several things orthodontists can do without surgery to affect facial profile. If the jaw is too far back, orthodontists can advance it to give the chin more projection. If the mid-face is too far back, such as with an underbite, an orthodontist can adjust the upper jaw so that it grows forward, giving the mid-face a little more projection and bringing the jaws in line with each other and with the skull.

We can make even more drastic changes with orthodontic surgery. Patients with "gummy" smiles, for instance, are often suffering from an over-eruption of front teeth, in which the teeth have grown downward too far, bringing the gums with them. To correct this, orthodontists can move the teeth back to a more ideal position, bringing the jaws into harmony. The gum line will naturally follow the teeth, resulting in a smile that shows much less gum. If needed, the patient can also undergo orthognathic (corrective jaw) surgery, which involves moving the whole jaw up so that the front teeth aren't excessively lower down.

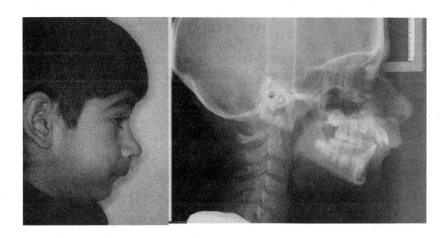

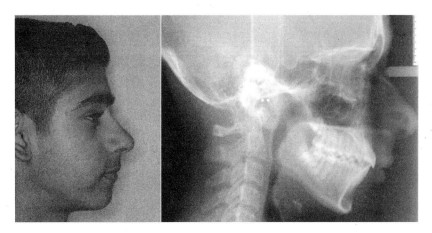

Notice the dramatic change in the patient's profile due to orthodontic treatment.

We can also take care of the reverse, where the teeth show very little when the patient smiles because the upper jaw is so high up. In most of these cases, the teeth can be moved down orthodontically, though some more severe cases may require surgery.

TREATING TMJ PAIN

A lot of the time, TMJ—*temporomandibular joint*, or simply the *jaw joint*—problems are caused by a number of problems, but one of the biggest factors is the patient's parafunctional habits: mouth/jaw habits apart from chewing, such as clenching or grinding.

When you have a poor bite, these parafunctional habits can cause much more harm. Grinding and clenching will have far more impact on the condition of the teeth and may lead to TMJ issues. While patients with a poor bite may not have TMJ issues, they are more likely to suffer from them, especially if they suffer from parafunctional habits.

ADVANCEMENTS IN TOOTH MOVEMENT

Since the early 2000s, the use of temporary anchorage devices, also known as TADs or TOADS (temporary [orthodontic] anchorage devices), has made moving teeth much easier and much less cumbersome for patients.

In the past, orthodontists would need to use external anchorage devices to move teeth, like headgear or face masks, or they'd have to pull on other teeth, which could lead to unintentional movement of the anchor teeth. With TADs, however, you can insert the small, screw-like device in the jawbone and move the teeth just by anchoring them to it.

If a tooth needs massive restoration, such as a root canal and crown, an orthodontist may recommend removing the tooth and closing the space with a TAD instead of going through the restoration process.

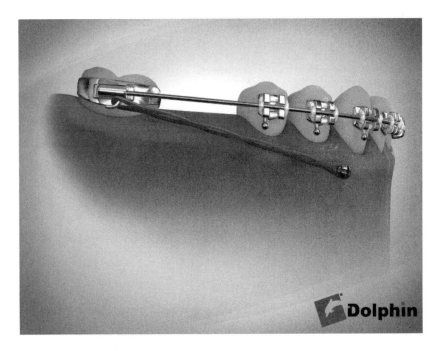

I've had several cases where patients thought they needed implants, and we were able to close the space with TADs instead. Several adults a year come for orthodontic treatment because of their bite before getting an implant, and in many of those cases, we were able to close that space instead. Kids will also visit with missing teeth and a recommendation from their dentist that they get an implant when they're older, maybe around seventeen or eighteen. But just as with the adults, there's a strong likelihood that we can close that space with TADs, and the child wouldn't need to worry about implants down the road.

Orthodontic Realities

EXTRACTION MAY BE THE BEST OPTION

Even with healthy teeth, extractions are sometimes necessary and may even be the best thing you can do for your mouth.

Once a person turns six or seven, and the first molars erupt in the mouth, the spacing of the teeth in the jaw is pretty much set, even though the jaw and body will continue to grow. So, from there on out, it's a question of how large or small the new, permanent teeth will be in relation to the jaw. As the teeth erupt, they'll either all be able to fit in the jaw, or they won't.

In a lot of cases, you just can't fit all the teeth in the jaw because there's too much tooth mass, which leaves you with two options: shaving down teeth to make them thinner, or extracting teeth to create more space within the jaw.

The reason for this overcrowding typically has to do with the size of the jaw and the size of the teeth not matching up. If teeth are trying to squeeze into the jaw, and there's not enough space in the bone, the teeth will naturally push to the outer edges, making them more susceptible to gum and bone recession, and periodontal problems. Such overcrowding also makes the mouth a lot more unstable. As the teeth crowd up, they automatically receive more pressure from the lips and cheeks, which want to push them back in.

Of course, the reverse can be true as well. If the teeth grow too far inward, it can create too much pressure on the tongue, causing it to push the teeth back out in a way that can result in awkward angling and gaps. This can also happen when a patient has a very large tongue. In most people, the teeth will erupt into a position that is at equilibrium (in balance) between the cheeks, lips, and tongue.

Ideally, the teeth should grow in a way that keeps them in an ideal position not only within the bone, soft tissue, and gums, but also between the tongue, lips, and cheeks to achieve a natural equilibrium. This will create a more stable result over the long term. Sometimes, this harmonious ideal can only be achieved with extraction.

THE LIMITATIONS OF JAW EXPANSION

There's a common misconception that expanding the jaw is better than extraction for relieving overcrowded teeth, but there are a few limitations to this approach. First, the lower jaw is made of a single, solid bone and cannot be expanded. You can move the teeth outward to expand the arch of teeth. In doing so you will gain approximately 1 mm of arch length space for every 3 mm of expansion.[12] This is not a very good ratio. The other problem is that the teeth are healthiest sitting in the middle of the bone, not on the outer edges of the bone.

The second principle one must consider is that of a coordinated upper and lower jaw. While the upper jaw can be expanded during the growing years, it still needs to coordinate with the lower jaw (which cannot be expanded). For example, if the upper jaw is 4 mm too narrow to coordinate with the lower jaw, then expanding the upper jaw by 4 mm would be advisable, but as studies have shown, this will only gain 1–2 mm of extra arch length in the upper arch.[13] Sometimes teeth just have to be extracted in order for them to all fit within the bone structures. It could be that the teeth are overcrowded, but the upper jaw is already expanded as far as it will go, or it's already in harmony with the lower jaw, which can't be expanded.

---

12   Nicholas Germane DMD et al., "Increase in arch perimeter due to orthodontic expansion," *AJO-DO* 100, no. 5 (November 1991): 421-27, https://doi.org/10.1016/0889-5406(91)70081-7.

13   Ibid.

Even when expansion is performed to help reduce overcrowding, it doesn't create a lot of space. For example, a typical result for expansions is about 1 mm of arch length for every 3 mm of expansion. A typical expansion is anywhere from 6 to 10 mm, so the most you can expect to get is around 3 mm of extra arch length—about the height of two stacked pennies.

Of course, you can increase that space by shaving teeth through a process called *interproximal reduction*. This is much more effective at gaining arch length than expansion. If you were to shave half a millimeter off each of your front eight teeth (a very safe amount of enamel reduction), you could gain another 4 mm of space. But sometimes even that isn't enough to relieve crowded teeth. To gain 4mm of arch length through expansion, you would need approximately 12 mm of expansion. That's a lot of expansion to the upper arch, and it still needs to be coordinated with the lower arch.

With tooth extraction, however, you can quickly gain anywhere between 14 mm and 16 mm of extra space within the jaw simply by removing two teeth.

SPEECH IMPEDIMENTS: EXPANSION IS NOT ALWAYS AN INSTANT FIX

Even though I spoke earlier in this chapter about speech impediments and how the skeletal structure of the mouth can influence them, expanding the palate and bringing the bite closer to the ideal is often only the beginning. The adjustment may help improve speech and correct the discrepancy so they're able to make sounds easier, but patients may still need speech therapy.

WE'RE NOT PLASTIC SURGEONS

Although orthodontists can affect the aesthetics of a smile and even improve lip posture and profile, we still can't make a person look radically different. Instead, the changes in facial appearance are going to be more subtle. The major changes are mainly seen in the patient's smile. The soft tissue of the lips, cheeks, chin, and nose are not changed.

The teeth and smile could look totally different, but when it comes to creating facial harmony, the patient is inevitably going to come out of it looking pretty much like the same person.

ORTHODONTICS IS NOT ONE-SIZE-FITS-ALL

Even though advertising and the media may make it seem as though teeth can be perfected in no time and with the same, simple procedures, this just isn't true. Orthodontics and dentistry in general are not one-size-fits-all. There are "procedures" that advertise straight teeth in as little as six months. These procedures are mainly touted by general dentists and there is nothing magical or special about these treatments. Any orthodontist can straighten the front teeth in six months. What the advertisers fail to mention is that the bite and jaw relationships are not addressed in these procedures. The complexity of most cases comes from trying to achieve a good bite and establish the proper relationships between the teeth and jaws and create a good facial balance.

I have many patients ask for certain treatment, such as Invisalign or expanders, and when I don't recommend it, they want to know why. Other patients may want their teeth straightened, but they don't want extractions, because none of their friends who had their teeth straightened needed it. I try to tell all my patients that, simply put, we're all unique. Braces or expanders may have one effect on one person and a different effect on another, so we can't always apply the same treatment to every patient.

Chapter 2 Summary

- In some cases, just straightening out the front teeth may actually take a bite from bad to worse.

- Correcting a bite is often far more complex than just putting on braces and often takes much longer than six months to complete.

- An ideal functional bite leads to a cleaner mouth, a more aesthetically pleasing smile, healthier jaw joints, a more balanced profile, and good chewing and speech functions.

- Bite complications can affect speech, making it difficult to pronounce certain sounds, such as *t*, *n*, and *d*, or causing an audible hissing effect on sibilant sounds such as *s* and *z*.

- Orthodontic treatment can improve self-esteem and confidence, and help patients engage and participate in every aspect of their life, potentially including their job prospects.

- Orthodontic treatment has been shown to help with sleep apnea, a condition some studies have linked to ADHD.

- Even with healthy teeth, extractions are sometimes necessary, especially when it comes to overcrowding.

- The upper jaw can be expanded, but the lower jaw cannot—it can only be repositioned.

- The same procedure will work differently for each patient. There is no one-size-fits-all treatment that provides the same results every time.

CHAPTER 3

Facial Beauty and the Science of Cephalometry

Most patients and parents of patients who come in for orthodontic treatment are hoping to look better and have a better-looking smile. And that's great! That's what orthodontists do. The disconnect often occurs in our respective definitions of "better-looking."

A lot of patients already have a pretty good idea of how they want their teeth to look when they're finished with treatment, but they don't necessarily understand all the details that go into getting their teeth into that position. Sometimes their ideals are a little unrealistic, or they don't have the facial or jaw structure to create the smile

43

they want, or they don't have the right size or shape to their teeth. That is, if a person was born with very small or misshapen teeth, there may limitations on what we can achieve orthodontically. Ultimately, there are just some things that we, as orthodontists, cannot change.

This may be surprising, especially when you watch some of these "extreme makeover" shows, where people who once had smiles that would suit a retired pirate are suddenly flashing superstar grins. Most people don't realize many of these patients get a mouthful of crowns and veneers. While this a quick solution to crooked, missing, or broken-down teeth, they eventually must replace these restorations every ten to fifteen years down the road. This can be very expensive over time, and unlike orthodontics, these restorations don't last forever.

THE SCIENCE OF CEPHALOMETRICS

When orthodontists think about how to move a patient's teeth into their ideal final position, they often use cephalometrics in the treatment planning process.

Cephalometry, or the measurement and study of the proportions of the head and face, is a study that stems from the turn of the twentieth century and the invention of the cephalogram, which is basically a precise x-ray of the head.

Even though orthodontics already existed by this time, the study of cephalometry wasn't widely used by the profession. Instead, early orthodontists focused on achieving the ideal bite and weren't really paying attention to the facial profile and tooth placement in the bone.

There was also a philosophy at the time that teeth didn't need to be extracted and instead, they could be lined up to achieve the ideal bite regardless of jaw structure or angulation of the teeth in the bone. The orthodontists believed if they could just straighten the teeth and achieve an ideal bite, then everything else—including facial aesthetics and tooth position in the bone—would take care of itself.

It wasn't until the middle of the twentieth century that orthodontists realized this just wasn't the case. Pioneers such as Dr. Charles Henry Tweed in the United States, and Dr. Percy Raymond Begg in Australia began to challenge orthodontics' nonextraction philosophy, pointing out the more stable outcomes from extractions and also the improved aesthetic results.

Tweed and Begg discovered that as hard as orthodontists worked to create an ideal bite, if the results were out of balance in the mouth then the teeth and tissues would eventually overcome a doctor's final results and move back to a position of equilibrium. The soft tissues of the muscles within the lips and cheeks would cause the teeth to relapse into misalignment. With proper extraction, however, the teeth could remain aligned in a healthier and more aesthetic position.

With this revelation, orthodontists began looking into cephalometry as a way to identify and quantify the healthiest and most aesthetic position of the teeth. Research projects were launched to discover the measurements of ideal facial balance, and dozens of studies were made of what laypeople, dentists, and orthodontists considered to be the most aesthetically pleasing.

At first, these studies compared the ideal bite, profile, and facial aesthetic of hundreds of caucasian American patients, with what was considered nice "facial balance," and close to an ideal occlusion and thus establishing "norms." Many of these studies first used beauty contestants because these were judged to be close to an ideal that appealed to the masses. Surprisingly, many of the characteristics and cephalometric norms were very similar within all of the ethnicities whenever beauty contestants were used as the ideals. This finding is probably due to the heavy influence of western media like magazines, movies, and television. This beauty pageant influence has been seen in almost every study; it is probably true that these ideals established from the beauty contestants probably do not truly represent a cross-section of the people judging them.

Over the years, many more studies were done on non-beauty contestants of many different ethnicities. From Japanese, to Chinese, to Malaysians, to Northern Indians, to Southern Indians, and almost every other ethnic group around the globe. The studies evolved to include dozens of different ethnicities, developing norms for a wide range of ethnic groups and racial backgrounds.

For instance, researchers found that an ideal facial aesthetic for natives of India includes front teeth that angle outward just slightly more than the Caucasian norm, as well as jaws that tend to favor slightly flatter angles. In East Asian facial norms, the mid-face area is usually not as prominent as it is in caucasian groups.[14]

But regardless of race or ethnicity, all of the studies examining the normal or ideal cephalometric characteristics of an ethnicity favored good facial balance, mouths with very little crowding of the teeth, and a bite that was close to ideal, if not perfect. While some of the cephalometric measurements were almost identical between different ethnicities, some measurements were slightly different. As orthodontists use cephalometrics to evaluate a case during treatment planning, we must remember what Steiner said about the norms of his cephalometric study, that "these estimates are to be used as guides

---

14   S.R. Tippu et al., "Soft tissue cephalometric norms for orthognathic surgery in Indian adults," *International Journal of Oral and Maxillofacial Surgery* 36, no. 11, 1020; Fujio Miura, Naohiko Inoue, and Kazuo Suzuki, "Cephalometric standards for Japanese according to the Steiner analysis," *International Journal of Orthodontia and Dentistry for Children* 51, no. 4, 288-95; Jen Soh, Ming Tak Chew, and Hwee Bee Wong, "A comparative assessment of the perception of Chinese facial profile esthetics," *American Journal of Orthodontics and Dentofacial Orthopedics* 127, no. 6, 692-99.

and must be modified for individuals." Steiner believed that these estimates were useful but should be modified per individual and per ethnicity. I believe wholeheartedly with Steiner in that these "cephalometric norms" created for each ethnicity and race should be only used as a guide, not as a goal for treatment. Every patient is an individual, even within an ethnicity. Each presents with different facial characteristics, size and shape of their teeth and jaws, and should be evaluated based on their own morphology.

PROFILE CONVEXITY

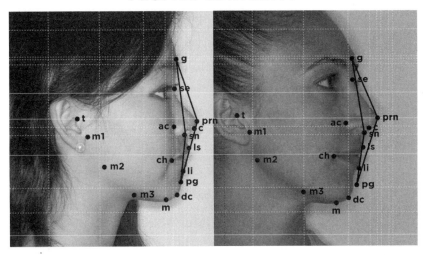

Both of these patients exhibit an ideal profile with very nice facial balance, yet their cephalometric characteristics are different. A reminder that cephalometric measurements are to used as a guide and not a goal of treatment.

CEPHALOMETRIC DIAGNOSIS: TWO-DIMENSIONAL MEASUREMENTS IN A THREE-DIMENSIONAL WORLD

In studying facial balance and beauty, researchers realized their results could only be viewed in two dimensions. However, people see each other in three dimensions, and fully animated; not static, two-dimensional profiles or frontal images, such as those used for measurements. Additionally, the measurements from these early studies tended to be somewhat inconsistent due to one other very important factor: beauty, as the old expression goes, is in the eye of the beholder. What one researcher found to be beautiful might not have been the same for another.

This doesn't mean that the measurements derived from these studies were invalid, but it does mean that orthodontists have to take any comparisons they do between a patient and a cephalometric ideal with a grain of salt and only make decisions about aesthetics based on a live clinical exam of the patient.

It's during this exam that the lip and tooth relationships can be evaluated from both a resting position as well as when the face is active and animated. That way the orthodontist can see important aspects, such as how patients' teeth relate to the lips as they smile and as they open and close their mouth, or how the soft tissues move across the hard support structures of jaw, cheek bone, and teeth.

At the same time, the diagnosis has to be interactive with the patient. The orthodontist may see an abnormality or an imbalance during the cephalometric analyses of x-rays and photographs, but the patient may not see the imbalance and may not share the same aesthetic values as the orthodontist or the cephalometric analysis.

With that in mind, however, it's the orthodontist's job to put the teeth in the healthiest position within the jaws, maximizing both function and aesthetics, so the final decision on treatment is usually a careful balance of both professional judgement and patient desires.

THE ROLE OF CEPHALOMETRICS IN ORTHODONTICS

When evaluating a patient for treatment, orthodontists don't necessarily treat to the norms. Even though that was the standard in the 1960s through the 1980s, treatments today look at cephalometric norms as more of a guide.

In evaluating a patient for the ideal bite and facial aesthetic, the orthodontist will likely use an overlay of that patient's cephalometric results over an image of cephalographic norms and look at where the patient and the norm deviate, how large the deviations may be, and whether or not those deviations are the cause of an imbalance, a bad bite, or poor aesthetics.

A patient who comes in with a large overbite, for example, may only see that his or her top front teeth stick out too far. But the angle and position of the teeth might not be the real cause of the problem. A cephalometric analysis may reveal that the lower jaw is too far back relative to the upper jaw. In that case, the issue would be a skeletal one that does not necessarily originate with the teeth. If this problem is caught during a patient's growing years, the jaw growth can be modified to help bring the patient's lower jaw forward, thus correcting the discrepancy between the upper and lower jaw and, in turn, correcting the bite. It is only through a cephalometric analysis that the orthodontist can determine where the root of the problem lies.

Fixing a jaw condition like this in an adult typically requires surgery, although there are some "camouflage" treatments that can move the teeth around in a way that helps mask the skeletal problem. These treatments don't necessarily address the core problem, but it can be an option for patients who don't want to go through surgery.

However, sometimes the overbite isn't due to jaw position, but instead is caused by overcrowding. The overcrowding may be causing the front teeth to stick out too far. The patient may notice the overbite and crowding but not realize how severely the teeth are angling outward. In these cases, we'll study the cephalogram and then point out exactly how severe the overbite is.

Once the overly protrusive angle of the front teeth is shown to patients on the cephalometric analysis, the patient can see the problem and get a quantifiable number as to how far off from normal they are. This is just one of the reasons why cephalometric analysis is so valuable: you can show patients not only how their teeth are currently sitting but also the difference relative to an ideal bite, so they can quantitatively appreciate the difference. This makes the process useful not only for diagnosing facial aesthetics but also for locating the true cause of a bad bite and educating patients on their treatment.

WHAT IS A CEPHALOMETRIC ANALYSIS?

What most patients see at first when evaluating their facial structure is the soft tissue. How do the lips, nose, chin, cheeks, and lower face appear in general and when smiling? An orthodontist will look a little deeper, using the patient's cephalometric norms to determine the following:

- Where the teeth sit in the alveolar, or tooth-bearing bones, of the jaws

- Where the jaws are positioned relative to the face and head

- Where the teeth sit relative to the chin, lips, nose, etc.

It's not until the orthodontist studies every aspect of the soft tissues, hard support structures, and other factors using cephalometrics that he or she can determine exactly how any skeletal and dental changes will affect the soft tissue and, ultimately, the overall aesthetic of the smile.

Even the smallest details, such as where the teeth sit in the bone relative to the lip and nose, have measurements and norms in orthodontics. Using these, orthodontists can determine why patients' smiles are too gummy, why their front teeth don't show enough when they smile, or why their smile is so narrow. Even the smallest detail can point to much larger issues. Of course, every patient's skeletal structure is unique in its own way, but by having these sets of norms, we can much more easily track down the source of problems and take steps to correct them.

For example, patients who ask about treatment for a jaw that sits too far to the right or left of their facial midline see the imbalance, but what they don't see is that the cause of this is the result of the upper jaw being too narrow—what orthodontists call a *posterior crossbite*. Although the issue is skeletal, it's expressed in the teeth and soft tissues of the face, as the jaw visibly sits to the left or right.

At our practice, we probably see about two or three patients a month with this offset jaw issue. Fortunately, most of the patients who come to us with this problem are pretty young, so we can treat it nonsurgically, expanding the upper jaw and bringing everything more in line. For adults, however, the condition is a little more difficult to treat and will usually require surgery to correct.

For this reason, I always tell the parents of young patients that it's much better for us to correct jaw issues now rather than waiting until our only option for fixing them is jaw surgery.

Adults that do wind up having the surgery, however, see it as a life-changing event. For most of them, they've dealt with their face and jaw being out of line for so long that they've become used to how it looks and feels. Once it's changed, they suddenly realize how much better-looking they are, how symmetrical their soft tissue becomes, and how far off their skeletal structure was. It's an exciting and dramatic difference.

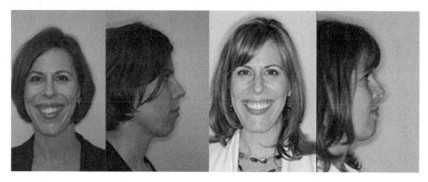

The photos on the left were taken before orthodontics and surgery. The two photos on the right were taken after treatment. Note the improvement in symmetry and profile.

VISIBLE DIFFERENCES

A lot of patients who come in for a complimentary examination are worried about the changes that may take place. Even if we're not talking about taking teeth out, they're worried about how they're going to look after the treatment is complete—how it will change their smile or affect their face. Their main concern is that a lot of this is irreversible.

To ease some of this worry, I, along with many other orthodontists, use computer models to show the patient approximately what they'll look like following treatment, keeping in mind that the computer-generated results and the actual results don't always look exactly the same. However, the computer images will show an approximation of the final result.

Additionally, we can show patients before and after images of similar patients who have had the same treatment and how it turned out. For instance, we can show them where the abnormalities were on other patients and how the end result brought their measurements more in line with the ideal cephalometric characteristics.

In the end, however, what I try to reiterate to patients is that there's a limit to how much we can move teeth in orthodontics. Even if we go to the outer limits, it's not going to dramatically change their face. For most patients, however, the changes are subtle and are mostly expressed in the smile.

CEPHALOMETRICS: COMMON MISUNDERSTANDINGS

There can be a lot of initial misunderstandings when it comes to orthodontics. Patients may come in believing their condition can be fixed one way, but cephalometric analysis of their case may show the problem is actually due to something completely different.

When it comes to overbites, for instance, many patients believe their teeth can be fixed just by bringing them back in line. But issues with the lower jaw, lower teeth, or other factors that aren't immediately visible may be the cause of the overbite. Studying the lateral cephalograph of a patient may show that a deep overbite is more skeletal in nature, or that it is a combination of both skeletal and dental components.

Ultimately, our job as orthodontists is to place the teeth in the healthiest position possible within the jaws while also trying to maximize function and aesthetics. And as doctors, we're going to take a more scientific approach to quantifying facial beauty and aesthetics. This way we can achieve more consistent results, but the problem remains that it's almost impossible to rigidly define aesthetics due to their highly subjective nature.

Chapter 3 Summary

- Orthodontists give you realistic expectations for a better-looking smile based on your facial and/or jaw structure.

- Cephalometrics is the measurement and study of the proportions of the head and face, and it's the science that orthodontists use to plan a patient's orthodontic treatment.

- Comparing a patient's cepholometric analysis to the normal values can help assess the severity of any skeletal and dental imbalances.

- Facial norms vary by ethnicity and are referred to when identifying a patient's ideal bite and facial aesthetics.

- Treatment decisions about a patient's ideal facial aesthetics should only be based on a live clinical exam.

- Cephalometric analyses are used to assess the extent of skeletal and dental problems and to identify less obvious factors that may be contributing to the issue.

- A cephalometric analysis is what an orthodontist uses to study every aspect of a patient's facial soft tissue (lips, nose, chin, cheeks, etc.), hard support structures, and other factors to determine how any skeletal and dental changes will affect the overall aesthetic of the smile.

Starting Orthodontic Treatment (What Age Is Too Young?)

H ere are two of the most common questions I get regarding adolescent and child patients:

1. How can I tell if my child needs braces?

2. If my child does need braces, what is the best age to get them?

These are both good and important questions, but they're also not easy to answer. To understand why, we'll have to take a couple steps back and look at the broader picture.

AGES SEVEN TO EIGHT: IMPORTANCE OF THE FIRST ORTHODONTIC EXAM

To ensure the health of your child's mouth, it's important to have an orthodontic exam between ages seven and eight. At this age, about half of all the permanent teeth are starting to come in, as well as the patient's first molars; this allows an orthodontist to see how both the bite and spacing within the mouth are developing. There are a lot of things that parents can't see on their own, including potential issues with jaw alignment, impacted teeth, chips or fracturing of teeth, or permanent teeth that aren't erupting well as they emerge from the gums. But orthodontists can spot these issues pretty quickly, usually with a fifteen- to twenty-minute exam, a few pictures, and potentially an x-ray or two.

A lot of these potential issues can be addressed at an early age as well and can prevent them from getting worse over time as the remaining permanent teeth erupt. At the same time, there's also the important psychosocial aspect of the treatment—kids treated at younger ages are likely to have better-looking teeth as their remaining permanent teeth erupt and are less likely to deal with any social stigmas that may come with an awkward smile.

The psychosocial aspect is important—most kids would argue it's the most important reason for any kind of dental treatment— but the main benefit of early interceptive treatment is in preventing problems that could potentially become a lot worse down the road. Issues that are skeletal in nature, for instance, can be corrected early on, before braces may be needed.

A lot happens between ages eight and twelve. Kids grow tremendously, which means if a skeletal issue exists, problems will be magnified as the patient continues to grow. Moreover, if a skeletal issue is allowed to persist to age thirteen, it will most likely get worse, because the patient may only have two or three years of very limited growth left at that age. This leaves a very small window to try and correct a problem that has been growing for seven to ten years. By the age of twelve or thirteen, those issues may have become too difficult to correct through less invasive methods, and the patient will have to wait until they are fully grown, at age seventeen or eighteen (sometimes nineteen or twenty, for boys), before the condition can be corrected with jaw surgery.

CAUSES AND CONTRIBUTORS TO BAD BITES IN YOUNG PATIENTS

Since skeletal structure and tooth position grow rapidly before the age of twelve, it's easier to throw that growth off-balance. Concerns such as early (or late) baby tooth loss, crowded teeth, upper or lower jaw misalignment, and spacing issues causing the blockage of permanent teeth are all things that should be corrected early.

In addition, parafunctional habits such as thumb sucking, tongue thrusting, poor tongue posture, or other tongue habits can create a poor bite early on due to the unnatural or abnormal pressures exerted on the teeth. Sleep apnea, may also be caused by jaw abnormalities that restrict the airway.

BREAKING THE HABIT: FIXED HABIT-CORRECTION APPLIANCES

Oral habits such as thumb sucking and tongue thrusting can have a detrimental effect on the teeth, not to mention the psychosocial consequences of these habits on school children. Even though young children may be teased for these habits at school, studies have shown that parental intervention is only effective about 40 percent of the time. However, if the child is fitted with a fixed habit-correcting appliance, the success rate for quitting jumps to 65 percent. If parental intervention *and* a fixed habit-correcting appliance are used, the chance of breaking the oral habit moves up to 92 percent.

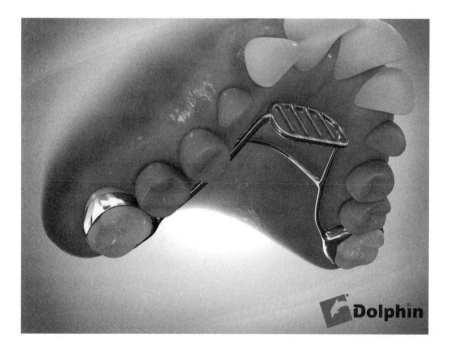

IMPACT AND TREATMENT OF COMMON BAD BITE CONDITIONS

LOSS OF BABY TEETH TOO EARLY (OR TOO LATE)

- **Cause**: Early baby tooth loss may be unintentional, such as a tooth being knocked out accidentally, or the tooth may be removed by a dentist due to trauma or cavities. For late tooth loss, the condition may be due to the permanent tooth coming in at a poor angle, thus failing to cause the natural loss of the baby tooth.

- **Impact**: The early or late loss of baby teeth can create spacing issues for permanent teeth because baby teeth serve as natural space maintainers. Typically, baby teeth are pushed out by the permanent tooth, which resorbs the root of the baby tooth and pushes the rest of the tooth out of the way. If the space isn't being held, or if a baby tooth is still there when the permanent tooth tries to emerge, then the permanent tooth can become stuck or emerge from the gums in an abnormal manner, such as to the outside of the gum or to the extreme inside. Orthodontists call this an *ectopic eruption*.

- **Treatment**: If an orthodontist sees this happening, they'll often recommend an extraction of the baby tooth if it hasn't fallen out yet. If a tooth falls out too early, an orthodontist might recommend a space maintainer, to prevent other teeth from drifting into the open spot until the permanent tooth grows in.

IMPROPER JAW ALIGNMENT

- **Cause**: One of the most common jaw misalignment problems we see is when the upper jaw doesn't grow wide enough to fit over the lower jaw. The fit should be like a shoebox lid, with the upper part slightly bigger than the lower part. This can be the result of genetics, obstructions in breathing, or thumb sucking, tongue thrusting, or other parafunctional habits that alter the natural growth of the jaw.

- **Impact**: If the upper jaw doesn't develop properly, the teeth of the upper jaw won't fit properly over the lower jaw teeth. This prevents proper chewing. To account for this, the patient will often unconsciously shift their jaw to one side or in various directions that allow them to chew better. Over time, this can cause the jaw to permanently shift to one side or the other, sometimes to an extreme.

- **Treatment**: If left untreated, this condition may require jaw surgery. However, it can be treated early on (age seven or eight is ideal) by widening the upper jaw and bringing the jaws into alignment with each other, resulting in a more symmetrical alignment of the jaw and face.

OVERBITE AND UNDERBITE

- **Cause**: Overbites, or what orthodontists call "overjet," are often the result of the lower jaw failing to grow far enough forward and the upper jaw growing too far forward. For underbites, the cause is just the opposite: The upper jaw fails to grow forward enough, and the lower jaw grows too far forward. Both conditions may be either hereditary or the result of a malformed jaw.

- **Impact**: An untreated overbite or underbite can affect chewing, speech, and breathing. In addition, there can be increased wear on the teeth due to the misalignment, which can increase the risk of tooth loss.

- **Treatment**: Interestingly, overbites can be corrected at older ages (twelve to fourteen years old) just as easily as they can be at a young age. However, underbites are best treated in two phases, with the first phase starting at age seven or eight, in order to take advantage of the jaw's growth before it reaches maturity.

ANTERIOR OPEN BITE

- **Cause**: An anterior open bite is when the front teeth do not overlap at all when the patient bites down. Normally, there is some overbite between the upper and lower incisors. When the anterior teeth do not meet or overlap, this could be due to several different factors. The most common causes are persistent parafunctional habits involving the tongue or fingers. Another cause could be skeletal in nature, as when the upper and lower jaws are growing in a divergent pattern.

- **Impact**: Repetitive and extended pressure against the front teeth—for example, with a habit—can cause the teeth to tilt outward, leaving a visible open gap between the upper and lower front teeth and often resulting in speech impediments. This also renders the anterior teeth nonfunctional and places all of the function on the posterior teeth. This can lead to excessive wear on the posterior teeth. In the long term, if the open bite is not treated, the posterior teeth can become completely worn down.

- **Treatment**: Children ages seven or eight can be treated with an appliance that helps them break the habit of exerting unnecessary pressure against the front teeth. They can also be given tongue exercises (also called *myofunctional exercises*) to do that will help prevent the habit.

There's a lot that can go wrong with the teeth and jaws at an early age, but fortunately, there's a lot that can be fixed at an early age as well—and with less invasive procedures than may be needed later on in adolescence or adulthood.

WHEN IS EARLY ORTHODONTIC TREATMENT NEEDED?

Statistically speaking, early orthodontic treatment in children ages seven or eight, and even up to ten, is only necessary in about 15 percent of the population. Most children don't need early treatment (also called *phase-one treatment*) and can be treated in a single, comprehensive phase once all their permanent teeth have erupted and the baby teeth are gone.

But even though the chances are low that your child may need early orthodontic treatment, the American Association of Orthodontists recommends all patients at age seven to get an orthodontic exam, even if it's just to rule them out of that 15 percent.

If a correction is needed at a young age, it's usually to correct crossbites, such as when the upper jaw needs to be expanded to fit properly over the lower jaw, or to correct other imbalances in jaw development. Occasionally we'll see young patients for early treatment who don't have a crossbite but do have very narrow upper and lower jaws. In these cases, the teeth are typically tipped in toward the tongue, making both jaws appear narrow. To treat this, an orthodontist would need to expand both the upper and lower arches, tilting the teeth upright and moving the teeth toward the lips and away from the tongue. This type of arch expansion mainly consists of uprighting the teeth within the bone. And in the lower jaw it is entirely tooth movement because the lower jaw cannot be expanded.

Because the lower jaw is a single, solid bone and cannot be expanded, "widening" it actually means moving the teeth outwards. The bone itself does not move. There are more options with the upper jaw because it is composed of two separate bones. These bones can be expanded to create a wider arch, which in turn gives more space for the tongue. This will help balance facial structure and aid conditions such as sleep apnea, which can be exacerbated by a narrow jaw.

WHEN EARLY ORTHODONTIC TREATMENT CAN WAIT: SEVERE OVERBITES

Although there are times, in the case of severe overbites, when orthodontic treatment is recommended at age seven or eight, waiting to correct the problem until the young patient has most of his or her permanent teeth may be just as effective as starting at an early age.

In a randomized clinical trial conducted in 2004, researchers found that a two-phase treatment of severe overbites/overjets (where the upper jaw extends more than 7mm beyond the lower jaw), starting in preadolescence and followed by a second phase during early adolescence, was no more clinically effective than a one-phase treatment of the condition during early adolescence.[15]

The study measured all of the changes involved, from

---

15 Tulloch et al., "Outcomes in a 2-phase randomized clinical trial of early class II treatment," *American Journal of Orthodontics and Dentofacial Orthopedics* 125, no. 6: 657–667.

skeletal or alignment to how the teeth came in, as well as the length and complexity of the treatment, and found that the two-phase approach was less efficient because it produced the same results as the one-phase but took twice as long and was much more complex.

However, some patients may still decide to do the two-phase treatment due to complications with sleep apnea (read more about sleep apnea later in this chapter) or for psychosocial reasons—if the child has a speech impediment due to the condition, is being teased at school, or is incredibly self-conscious, then the overbite can be treated earlier.

WHAT'S THE BEST AGE TO GET BRACES?

Every patient is different, and because of that, there's no straightforward answer to the best age for getting braces. As a rule of thumb, the vast majority of kids who need braces will get them once all of their permanent teeth have erupted. That age, however, can vary from as young as nine-and-a-half up to sixteen years old, although most children have all of their permanent teeth by age twelve, which is usually around seventh grade.

There are kids on both sides of the age curve, of course, but it's rare (only about 10 percent of children) for braces to be recommended before all of a child's permanent teeth have come in. Treatment in the mixed dentition (half baby teeth, half adult teeth) phase is usually only recommended for special cases where there may be issues that need to be corrected as soon as possible and where, if left untreated, the severity of the problem would get much worse. For these patients, two phases of treatment will most likely be needed: one around age seven or nine, and a second at age twelve or thirteen, once all of the permanent teeth erupt.

OPTIONS FOR BRACES

Braces and other dental appliances are discussed in further depth in chapter 5, but young patients should know that there are options for making braces much less visible than they were even five years ago.

Stainless steel braces: Those of us who had their braces twenty, thirty, or forty years ago remember them as bulky railroad tracks that could be seen from fifty yards away. But today's stainless steel braces are much smaller and much less visible, and they also come with a fun array of elastic tie color options that span the spectrum.

Clear braces: These braces began as a plastic composite in the early 1980s and have since been developed using a crystal-clear or tooth-colored monocrystalline or polycrystalline ceramic. These braces are very aesthetically pleasing and hard to notice—even the metal wires come with the option of a tooth-colored coating that makes them less visible. The new polycrystalline brackets are stronger, which means less fracturing or breakage of the braces. These new ceramic braces function just like metal braces and are just as durable. Some of them, like the braces manufactured by 3M Unitek, are made with a patented design that allows them to be removed from the teeth very easily, thus reducing much of the risk associated with ceramic brackets. In the past, many ceramic brackets were difficult to remove from the teeth and, in some rare cases, caused enamel fractures as they were removed.

No matter the type of braces you choose, the technology for these appliances has improved to the point where they are smaller, more efficient, and safer. Because they are smaller, they are more aesthetic, less noticeable, and harder to see in pictures. The less conspicuous nature of braces today make them much easier for kids (and adults!) to wear without feeling self-conscious.

EARLY INTERCEPTION TOOTH EXTRACTIONS

About 6.4 million people, or 2 percent of the US population, are diagnosed with impacted upper canines, which are the most commonly impacted teeth. However, if an orthodontist is able to identify that a permanent canine is coming in abnormally before the baby canine tooth falls out, then early extraction of the baby canine can help "normalize" the position of the permanent canine. In fact, this method of extraction in children before the age of eleven has been shown to be more than 75 percent effective.[16]

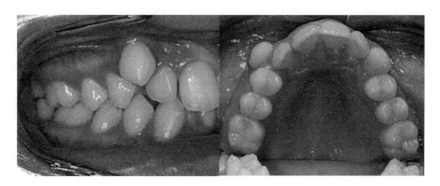

Extracting baby teeth can be a great interceptive technique and is one of the first lines of defense when it comes to treatment options and proactively preparing a young patient's teeth for a healthy, uncrowded

---

16   Manne et al., "Impacted Canines: Etiology, Diagnosis, and Orthodontic Management." *Journal of Pharmacy & Bioallied Sciences* 4, no.2 (2012): S234–S238.

mouth down the road. It can help avoid braces, or if braces are still recommended, the process will help expedite the braces-wearing process and make it more effective.

DIAGNOSING ECTOPICALLY ERUPTING CANINES IN YOUNG PATIENTS

To determine if a young patient's canines are coming in ectopically, or abnormally, an orthodontist will look at both the baby and permanent teeth in a few different ways:

Palpation of the canine eminence: During a young patient's intraoral exam, an orthodontist will palpate the area just above the baby canine tooth, which is called the *canine eminence*. If he or she feels the permanent canine, then it will likely come in normally. If he or she can't feel it, then that could be an indication of that the canine is not coming in properly.

Visual confirmation: Another indication that a canine could be erupting ectopically is if the front tooth next to it (the maxillary lateral incisor) is out of its normal position. If it is, this could also indicate an abnormally emerging tooth pushing the incisor out of position.

Panoramic x-ray: As a standard of care, panoramic x-rays are routinely taken during the exam and during treatment to evaluate all of the permanent teeth. These x-rays will show how the canine is erupting and are a must before any treatment decisions can be made.

Asymmetry is the other thing an orthodontist looks for when doing an exam of a patient before the age of eleven. If he or she can feel the permanent canine coming in on one side and not on the other, this would be an indication that the teeth might not be coming in correctly. The orthodontist will likely recommend an x-ray to confirm.

If the problem is caught before age thirteen and the baby tooth is extracted, young patients are more likely to avoid impaction (teeth that fail to erupt) of the permanent canines, as well as keep the adjacent teeth healthy. However, if the possible impaction isn't caught in time, the emerging canine may erupt abnormally or, in the worst-case scenario, erupt into the adjacent incisor and resorb the incisor's root, which may result in the loss of that tooth.

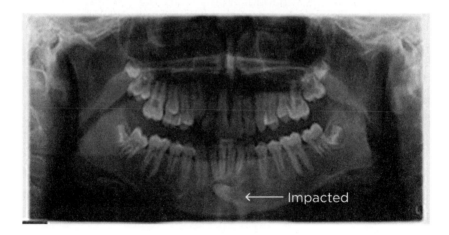

←——— Impacted

COMPLICATIONS WITH THE ERUPTING SECOND MOLAR

Another commonly impacted tooth is the second molar, which usually comes in at the age of twelve. Although not as common as canine tooth impaction, the second molar can come in at an angle and shove into the first molar, causing impaction; or it may not have enough room to erupt at all due to tooth crowding.

In the case of crowding, sometimes the bicuspid (the tooth right behind the canine—also called the first or second premolar) needs to be extracted in order to make room. However, if impaction is the problem, an orthodontist may recommend *expose and bond* surgery, which involves removing the tissue above the emerging molar and attaching a chain to tow it into place and help it emerge normally.

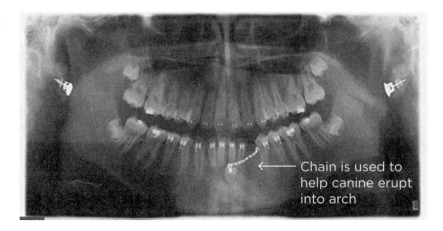

Chain is used to help canine erupt into arch

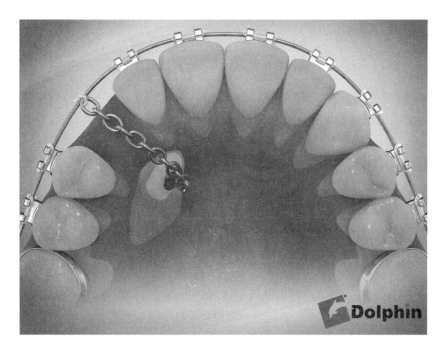

If a patient opts for the expose and bond procedure, he or she will likely need braces and see the orthodontist every four to six weeks for the next several months to have the chain on the second molar tightened and the progress of the emerging tooth evaluated.

CONGENITALLY MISSING TEETH

During a young patient's first exam, another possible issue that orthodontists look for is congenitally missing teeth. If caught early enough, young patients can often avoid having to replace those missing teeth at a later age by extracting certain baby teeth early on. This is especially true in the case of missing lower second bicuspids (the second tooth back from the canine), which is the second most commonly missing tooth after the wisdom teeth.

In my office, I see about two to three cases a year where patients are missing their permanent lower second bicuspids, which is indicated by a panoramic x-ray. In these cases, if we catch it early enough, and if the jaw seems to be a little too crowded, I often recommend extracting the baby tooth and allowing the molars to drift forward and close the space. Usually this is only recommended in cases that present with certain characteristics, like crowding or severe protrusion, where we are most likely going to extract teeth anyway.

If this extraction of the baby tooth is done at a young age—between seven and eight—the permanent molar behind the baby tooth will drift forward into place fairly quickly over the course of three to four years. However, if the problem isn't diagnosed until age twelve or thirteen, there will not be sufficient time to allow the permanent molar to drift forward on its own. In these cases, extracting the baby teeth may only be recommended if the jaw is very crowded or has excessive protrusion. But in cases where there is very little crowding and/or protrusion, moving the molar forward to close the space may be difficult and may require the use of an anchorage device like a TAD, which I covered previously in Chapter 2.

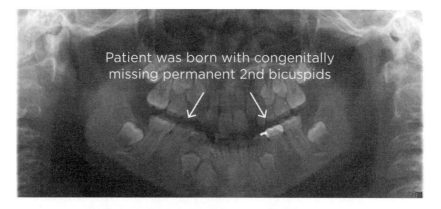

Patient was born with congenitally missing permanent 2nd bicuspids

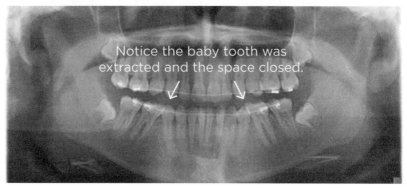

Notice the baby tooth was extracted and the space closed.

SLEEP APNEA

Another reason for early orthodontic treatment in young patients is sleep apnea. While there are causes for sleep apnea that aren't related to the mouth and throat structure, a lot of the time this condition can be treated by making adjustments to the jaw. In the majority of sleep apnea cases in children, there is some part of the tissues in the throat or nasal area that is causing the airway to become obstructed during sleeping. Changing the size and position of the jaws can have a dramatic effect on keeping the airway open during sleep. Thus, orthodontists are in a prime position not only to uncover the sleep apnea but also to effect the change needed to correct the condition.

Depending on the patient's condition, sleep apnea can be treated by expanding the upper jaw, expanding the dental arch on the lower jaw, and/or advancing the lower jaw. All of these steps tend to open up the airway, allowing for improved air flow and positively affecting—or even curing—the patient's sleep apnea.

As for diagnosing sleep apnea, orthodontists are adept at noticing the signs and symptoms of the condition. We also routinely take lateral cephalograms (x-rays) that can often reveal areas of the airway that are constricted and may become obstructed during sleep. If sleep apnea is suspected, the orthodontist may ask the patient questions from the Epworth sleepiness scale to determine if this is an issue. If so, then he or she may recommend that the patient have a sleep test done and have a formal diagnosis by a medical doctor before proceeding with treatment.

As orthodontists, the problem that we often run into with parents is that they don't think an orthodontic exam is necessary until kids have lost most, if not all, of their baby teeth. However, as the earlier issues show, an early exam is one of the best things you can do for your child's oral health. Ideally, every child should have an orthodontic exam between the ages of seven and eight, even if it's just to determine that they *don't* need any kind of treatment before all their permanent teeth are in.

Chapter 4 Summary

- A child should see an orthodontist for the first time between ages seven and eight. If there are any potential emerging issues, the orthodontist can usually spot these with a fifteen- to twenty-minute exam, a few pictures, and potentially an x-ray or two. Statistically, only about 15 percent of children this age need treatment, but it's wise to rule them out of that 15 percent as early as possible.

- The human body rapidly grows between ages eight and twelve. The earlier an issue is identified, the earlier it can be fixed and potential problems avoided down the road. By the age of twelve or thirteen, these issues may become too difficult to correct through less invasive methods, and the patient may have to wait until they're fully grown (age seventeen, eighteen, or even twenty, when it comes to males) to correct the issue with jaw surgery.

- Skeletal structure and tooth position can be thrown off more easily during the early growth years. Poor bite issues can be caused by habits such as thumb sucking, poor tongue posture, or other unnatural or abnormal pressures exerted on the teeth.

- Early or late loss of baby teeth, improper jaw alignment, overjet, underbite, or an anterior open bite can also cause poor bite conditions in children.

- Most children don't need early treatment—also known as *phase-one treatment*. Many can be treated in a single, comprehensive phase once all of their permanent teeth have erupted.

- If a child's permanent canine is coming in abnormally, extraction of the baby canine is 75 percent effective in normalizing the position of the permanent canine. If caught before the age of thirteen, young patients are more likely to avoid impaction of their permanent teeth.

- An orthodontist can determine if a permanent canine is coming in abnormally by palpating the area and doing a panoramic x-ray.

Braces, Functional Appliances, Removable Appliances

There are basically two types of appliances used in orthodontic treatment today: *orthodontic appliances* and *orthopedic appliances*. Both share the same Greek word *orthos*, which means "straight, upright, or correct," but they affect two very different, and specific, areas of the mouth.

Orthodontic appliances derive from the Greek word *odontos*, which means "teeth." Orthodontic appliances correct the teeth, as opposed to the bone around the teeth. **Orthopedic appliances** modify the growth of bones and thus modify the relationships of the skull to the upper and lower jaws.

While the word *orthopedic* is often associated with children (and the Greek word *paidion* actually does mean "child"), a 1741 work by French physician Nicolas Andry de Bois-Regard titled *Orthopaedia* led to the word *orthopedics* encompassing all treatments involving the musculoskeletal system.

THE DIFFERENCE BETWEEN ORTHODONTIC AND ORTHOPEDIC APPLIANCES

In use, orthodontic appliances are designed to deliver a specific amount of force over time: typically, a lighter, constant force (about fifty to a hundred grams of force) that results in tooth movement within the bones. These appliances tend to be smaller and lighter than orthopedic devices, and the forces they apply are usually continual, putting pressure on a certain tooth or group of teeth twenty-four hours a day, such as the way braces put pressure on your teeth around the clock. This pressure then forces the tooth and its supporting periodontal ligament to move, causing the bone in the area to remodel.

Imagine it like a spoon moving through a particularly thick batter. As the spoon moves forward, the batter moves out of the way in front of it and fills in the void behind it, where the spoon used to be. The teeth are like the spoon—as they move forward through the trough of the jaw bone, the bone in front of the tooth is torn down and rebuilt immediately behind it. The speed of this process of bone metabolism is what determines how fast the teeth move during orthodontic treatment. In adults, this process is usually slower than in children.

Orthopedic devices, on the other hand, are designed to affect the bone and therefore tend to use much greater forces than orthodontic devices—between 300 and 500 grams of force, for comparison. Additionally, because many orthopedic devices apply that force via the teeth, the use of an orthopedic device often results in both skeletal and dental movement. These forces are directed at the sutures of the bones, where the growth of the bones occurs, and when larger forces are applied to these areas, there is a modification to the growth of these bones.

A BRIEF HISTORY OF ORTHODONTIC APPLIANCES

Edgewise appliances are considered to be the forerunner of today's modern braces and brackets that most patients wear today. Invented by Dr. Edward Angle in the 1920s, Edgewise appliances consist of a metal bracket welded to a band, which is then wrapped entirely around the tooth. Rectangular arch wires are then run through the brackets to engage them and move the teeth three-dimensionally.

To activate the Edgewise device, the arch wire is bent in such a way that, as the wire returns to its original shape, it engages the bracket and pulls the tooth along with it, straightening both the tooth and the arch. The Edgewise appliance grew to become a standard in orthodontic care and remained such until the 1960s.

A lot has changed since the early 1900's. For Angle and his contemporaries, "braces" consisted of full bands, or rings, that went around every tooth in movement. Gold and silver were the metals most commonly used to make these bands, in addition to platinum, steel, wood, ivory, zinc, and copper to form hooks and other auxiliaries. However, these materials were not ideal. Although easy to mold and shape into bands, gold and silver were incredibly expensive. Additionally, these metals are soft, and therefore distorted easily, requiring frequent appointments and refitting. And, as far as esthetics, you can probably imagine the amount of metal that was visible when a patient smiled!

Many of the shortcomings of these early braces were addressed in the late 1950s when stainless steel became the material of choice for orthodontic appliances. Stainless steel was still easily formed into the shapes necessary for orthodontic appliances and wires, but, unlike its gold and silver predecessors, predictably held its shape and could be regularly bent to facilitate orthodontic movement at a fraction of the cost.

However, thanks in large part to advances in aerospace and automobile engineering, orthodontics began integrating advanced metal alloys into its appliances, and by the 1970s, many of the orthodontics we use today were being developed.

At the forefront of this evolution was Dr. Lawrence Andrews, who, in the 1970s, authored the landmark paper "Six Keys to Normal (Optimal) Occlusion," wherein he detailed how an ideal bite should look and how the teeth should naturally fit together.[17]

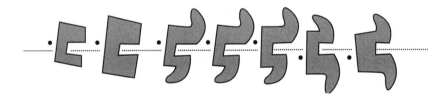

Andrews wrote this paper after studying and measuring approximately 120 cases that were considered to be "ideal," either because they were naturally ideal or because an orthodontic treatment brought them to an ideal state. Taking what he'd learned from these cases, he then developed a bracket system that incorporated all the

---

17   Lawrence Andrews, "The Six Keys to Normal (Optimal) Occlusion," *American Journal of Orthodontics and Dentofacial Orthopedics* (1972): 296–309.

ideal characteristics for each tooth in the mouth, meaning that each bracket for each tooth reflected exactly how that tooth should sit. The result is what we call the Straight-Wire Appliance.

Theoretically, an orthodontist could cement the brackets into their ideal positions and then place the wire in the brackets' slots. The wire would them move the teeth into the ideal position and bite, with no wire bending required.

However, one has to keep in mind that the pre-adjusted appliance was based on the average of those 120 sets of teeth, and while most patients will benefit from moving the teeth as close to average as possible, for those patients that slightly differ from average, the orthodontist has to make adjustments to the appliance. For instance, the orthodontist may have to bend wires or place brackets in slightly different positions, or use adjunct appliances like interarch elastics, headgear, or another appliance that works in conjunction with the braces.

Over time, these variances proved that not every patient could achieve an ideal bite with the Straight-Wire Appliance and that the device often needed modification to achieve ideal results. In response to this, several other orthodontists developed their version of the pre-adjusted Straight-Wire Appliance, including Drs. Roth, Ricketts, Burstone, Cetlin, McLaughlin, Bennet, and Trevisi.

Today, the Straight-Wire Appliance continues to be developed, with improvements such as clear brackets made from ceramics, self-ligating brackets (braces that use a clip to hold the wire in the bracket instead of elastics), and lingual brackets, which often use computerized placement to position brackets ideally on the tongue side of the teeth instead of the traditional, lip-facing side.

Lingual braces are currently at the forefront of orthodontic appliances. As of 2017, less than two percent of orthodontists use computerized placement of the brackets, choosing instead to rely on personal and professional experience to place the brackets ideally on the teeth.

Apart from these appliances, the invention of a way to bond the brackets directly to the teeth instead of welding the brackets to tooth-wrapping bands was a significant advancement in orthodontics. Developed in the 1970s, this bonding method wasn't popular until the 1980s, but the difference in both effectiveness and aesthetics was significant.

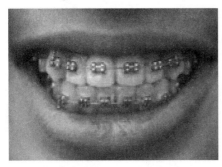

To bond the bracket to the tooth, the tooth enamel is lightly etched to create microscopic nooks and crannies, creating a rougher surface so that specialized cement can attach to it. The bracket, which is welded to a mesh pad, is pressed to the cement and cured in place using light to catalyze the reaction, a process that takes twenty to thirty seconds.

WHAT ORTHOPEDIC APPLIANCES ARE USED FOR

As we touched on earlier, orthopedic appliances are used when modifications need to be made to the bone—for what orthodontists call "skeletal discrepancies"—as opposed to the tooth.

For instance, in some patients, the lower jaw may be positioned too far back from the upper jaw, creating a large overjet, or "buckteeth." In other cases, the lower jaw may have grown too far forward from the upper jaw, creating an underbite.

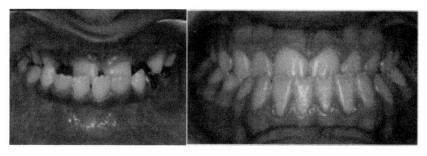

Both of these patients have had a lower jaw that has outgrown the upper jaw creating an underbite. Over time the lower jaw will continue to grow this way if the upper jaw is not expanded to fit with the lower jaw.

The width of the jaws can also cause complications. The upper jaw may be too narrow to fit with the lower jaw, creating what's called a crossbite in the back teeth. In these cases, patients often experience what's called a *functional shift*, where they can't bite down properly unless they shift their jaw to the right or left, changing the way their jaw functions to accommodate for their teeth not fitting together well enough to effectively chew.

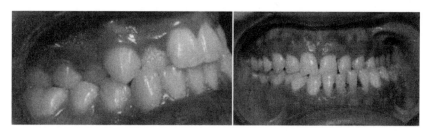

Both of these patients have a crossbite in the posterior teeth due to a narrow upper jaw. This can cause the lower jaw to have a functional shift to one side. Over time, the lower jaw will continue to grow this way if the upper jaw is not expanded and brought forward.

There are many variations on these conditions, of course, but these are the general skeletal discrepancies that orthopedic appliances are used to correct.

TREATING SKELETAL DISCREPANCIES

In general, there are three ways in which orthodontists can treat patients with skeletal discrepancies:

1. Dental camouflage

2. Orthognathic surgery

3. Orthopedic appliance therapy/growth modification

Which of these treatments is used typically depends largely on the severity of the skeletal discrepancy and the age of the patient.

DENTAL CAMOUFLAGE

Sometimes, a skeletal discrepancy will be camouflaged. This means that the discrepancy is small enough not to be noticeable, and just moving the teeth to an ideal bite may be the best alternative. In other words, it's an orthodontic (tooth-moving) treatment instead of a skeletal one, which means using a smaller, lighter orthodontic appliance instead of a larger orthopedic appliance. The downside to this option is that it usually requires extracting some teeth, and the end result may not be ideal—although it's often a huge improvement with good aesthetic results. This option is best for smaller skeletal discrepancies and for correcting bites when surgery is not an option.

ORTHOGNATHIC SURGERY

Orthognathic surgery is used to correct large skeletal discrepancies and to correct discrepancies in patients who are no longer growing.

For instance, if the lower jaw is set too far back and is just too small for the upper jaw, just taking out teeth and moving the upper front teeth back (an example of dental camouflage) may not be a viable option to bring it back into alignment: the lower jaw is just too far back and too small. This leaves surgery as the only alternative.

Although this option to correct patients' skeletal discrepancies aren't appealing to most, surgical results are often very effective. Ultimately, it creates an ideal finish, moving the teeth together into an ideal bite while also giving the jaws an ideal position relative to the rest of the face, which can help with the patient's overall appearance by making it more symmetrical.

There are some amazing changes that can be made with jaw surgery. It can affect a patient's overall well-being, not only improving their facial balance but also giving them better function overall, allowing them to chew better and have a more ideal bite, among other benefits. In some cases, it may even improve their sleep apnea.

ORTHOPEDIC APPLIANCE THERAPY/ GROWTH MODIFICATION

Lastly, the growth modification option is usually the best choice for patients who are still growing, as it often avoids the necessity for extractions or jaw surgery. In general, this option is used before the age of twelve or thirteen, aside from boys, who mature later in life than girls, and can sometimes be treated with growth modification into their mid-teens.

When it comes to growth modification, orthopedic appliances are generally designed using the teeth as anchors to transmit pressure to the underlying skeletal structure. Because this pressure is much stronger than the pressure used with orthodontic appliances, such as braces, they're often applied intermittently—between ten to twelve hours a day—instead of continuously.

However, the more these appliances are used, the bigger the impact; so, if they're worn for longer—say, fourteen to sixteen hours a day—they'll work better. Additionally, if the patient is going through a growth spurt, the appliance will also have more of an impact.

Depending on the type of discrepancy, different appliances may be recommended. For instance, if the upper jaw needs to move forward, such as with an underbite, the appliance will need to create a forward pull on the upper jaw, encouraging it to grow more in that direction.

This same approach, however, doesn't work for the lower jaw, as it's not structured the same way as the upper jaw. It has no sutures.

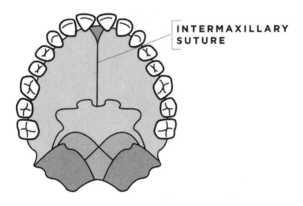

INTERMAXILLARY SUTURE

Upper (maxillary) jaw has a suture down the midline that allows it to be expanded before the suture closes in the late teenage years.

Structurally, your upper jaw is comprised of plates that can be encouraged to grow either forward or side-to-side while your skeletal system is still developing (typically before the age of thirteen). This growth takes place where the plates meet—the *sutures*—where bone is created to fill in the gap as the sutures are encouraged to move apart.

The lower jaw, however, is one solid bone, which means there are no sutures where the bone can be encouraged to grow or be expanded. However, though orthodontists are able to modify the lower jaw's *position*, we cannot change the shape or size of the lower jaw. If the lower jaw needs to be modified, an orthodontist can make it seem as though it has grown forward, but what has actually happened is that the lower jaw has simply been repositioned. This change takes place in the jaw joint in a shallow depression in the bone known as a *glenoid fossa*. There is permanent bone remodeling that takes place as the jaw is forced to function in a more forward position.

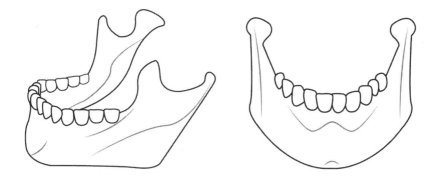

The lower jaw, the mandible, has no sutures and is one single solid bone. It has no capacity for expansion.

Once in place, orthopedic appliances work based on four factors:

1. **Force magnitude**: The amount of force applied while the appliance is in use.

2. **Force duration**: How long the appliance is used each day and over what period of time.

3. **Patient growth**: The appliances work best during the time of rapid growth.

4. **Timing**: The optimal time to use orthopedic appliances is at night, which is when the most growth of the human

body occurs; the best overall time is when the patient is in the prime growing years.

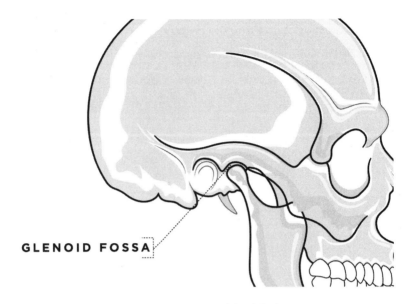

GLENOID FOSSA

The glenoid fossa is where the condyle of the lower jaw sits.

COMMON ORTHOPEDIC APPLIANCES

There are dozens of orthopedic appliances on the market, and while I don't go into all the nuances and variations of the different appliances in this book, I will discuss several of the most common devices:

- palatal expanders

- headgear

- protraction facemask

- chin cup appliance

PALATAL EXPANDERS

The palatal expander is probably the most common orthopedic device we use. The appliance is typically cemented onto the back teeth and worn for twenty-four hours a day, with certain types offering continual activation. Others are activated by turning a screw, which is considered intermittent activation.

These appliances take advantage of the midline suture in the palate, which doesn't fuse into solid bone until the patient is done growing. These appliances can expand the upper jaw by 2–12 mm. For most patients, the upper jaw is over-expanded until it is 2–4 mm too wide for the lower jaw. Once the expander is removed, the upper jaw will constrict slightly and become the perfect width to fit with the lower jaw. The expansion is usually completed within the first two months, but the expander remains in the mouth until the bone is completely healed and has filled in the area where the expansion occurred. This will usually take another four to five months, so the full length of treatment time with an expander is six to eight months.

HEADGEAR

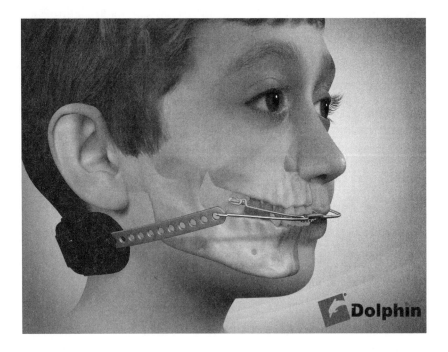

These appliances are usually used to correct both the overlapping of the upper teeth over the lower teeth, what orthodontists call an *overjet*, and overbites, which occur when the upper teeth stick out significantly beyond the lower teeth.

There are two types of headgear designed to correct this condition: occipital headgear, which moves the upper jaw back and up, and cervical headgear (as it wraps around the top of the neck, where the cervical vertebrae are located), which moves the upper jaw back and down. In either case, the headgear is designed with tubes that hook onto brackets placed on the molars. The molars are then used as anchorage to pull the upper jaw back and restrict its forward growth, allowing the lower jaw to grow forward and ultimately correct the overbite.

PROTRACTION FACEMASK

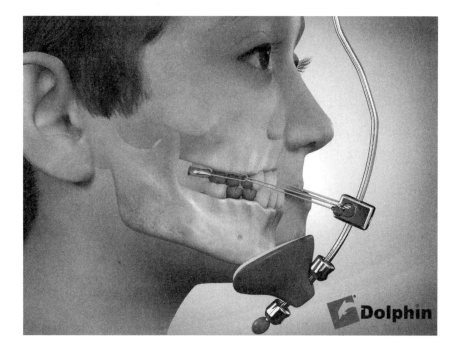

A protraction facemask, also called *reverse-pull headgear*, is worn on the front of the face and is typically used to correct underbites, which can occur when the mid-face isn't developing as quickly as the lower jaw, leaving it visibly "behind" the lower jaw. This device works best with younger patients, usually between the ages of seven and ten, although it can be used on older kids, up to age thirteen.

The device works by pulling the upper jaw forward using elastics, helping it stay in line with the lower jaw and bringing the entire face in line.

CHIN CUP APPLIANCE

This appliance is one of the older devices that's still in circulation today and is not seen as often as the devices mentioned earlier.

Although it was originally used to modify the growth of the lower jaw, we've since learned that it's very difficult, if not impossible, to alter the growth of the lower jaw. Instead, the chin cup device is used to help modify the position of the lower jaw and can be used in conjunction with orthodontic devices such as Invisalign.

FIXED FUNCTIONAL ORTHOPEDIC APPLIANCES

Fixed functional orthopedic appliances were developed in response to all the removable functional appliances that were found to be effective and beneficial, but were difficult to wear and difficult to get patient compliance with. The *Herbst* appliance was the first such device, followed by the *mandibular anterior repositioning appliance* (MARA); both were designed to be cemented onto the teeth with the goal of altering the patient's jaw function to an ideal position. Both devices cause changes in growth in the upper jaw and a repositioning effect in the lower jaw.

HERBST DEVICE

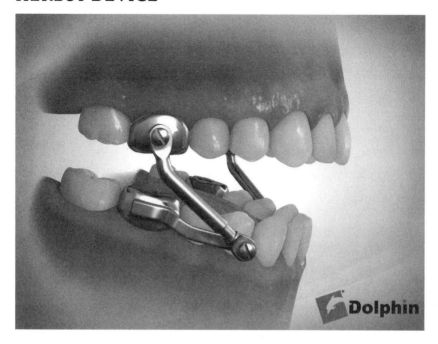

The Herbst device, developed by Dr. Herbst in 1934, is a fixed appliance designed to treat overbites. It uses two sliding metal rods attached to brackets on the upper molars and to two metal bars that run parallel to the lower back teeth. This system holds the lower jaw forward, eventually correcting the overbite. While it's always partially working to affect this adjustment, the Herbst appliance becomes 100 percent activated when the teeth are closed.

In the past, our practice used Herbst appliances quite a bit. More recently we have moved away from them due to their multiple moving parts and tendency to break a little more often than the MARA.

MARA

The MARA is also used to correct overbites and follows the same principle as the Herbst: it holds the jaw in the desired position, ideally moving the jaw into the correct bite by using a sliding elbow fitted in brackets attached to the upper molars. The lower molar is then fitted with a crown with a small "arm" projecting outward toward the cheek. As the patient bites down, the lower jaw has to move forward enough so that the elbow slips in front of the arm, allowing the patient to fully bite down.

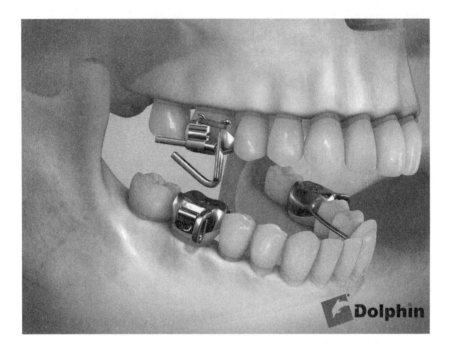

Because there's no direct connection between the upper and lower jaws, like the Herbst, the device is only 100 percent active when the mouth is closed.

COMMON ORTHODONTIC APPLIANCES

Orthodontic appliances are devices that apply pressure to a tooth or group of teeth in order to move them in a predetermined direction. Such appliances come in both fixed and removable forms.

Because orthodontic devices move the teeth—as opposed to modifying bone, as orthopedic devices do—they're designed to deliver a lighter, more continuous force. These appliances have high maximum elastic load, which means they can stretch or bend without breaking while also being able to move the tooth precisely, without unwanted movement. In other words, the appliance has a self-limiting force that, if worn for a long time without seeing an orthodontist, is not going to push the teeth out of the bone.

Additionally, orthodontic devices have an ease of insertion in the mouth and can withstand forces such as those created while chewing.

On a biological level, orthodontic devices should be able to produce tooth movement in the desired direction without interfering with speaking or chewing and without having deleterious effects to the teeth or bones (it shouldn't cause resorption of the teeth or damage the TMJ).

Of the two types of orthodontic appliances, fixed and removable, fixed appliances are probably the most well-known, and among them, braces are by far the most common.

BRACES

Braces are cemented onto the teeth and help translate the force from the arch wire to the tooth, moving the group of teeth in the desired direction. There are three main types of braces:

1. Tip-Edge

2. lingual

3. self-ligating brackets

TIP-EDGE

Tip-Edge braces, also known as Begg brackets, were a modification of the original Edgewise appliance, which we spoke of at the beginning of the chapter. Although they've fallen out of favor today, the Tip-Edge system designed with a modification of the bracket slot so that the tooth could be angled more, as opposed to the Edgewise, which simply allowed the tooth to slide along the arch wire and didn't allow for any angled adjustment.

When the Tip-Edge was developed by Drs. Begg and Kesling, a lot of orthodontists were doing four-bicuspid extractions in order to pull back the anterior, or front teeth, anchoring the front teeth to the posterior (back) teeth to draw them backward. By using Tip-Edge braces along with this procedure, the patient ultimately required less anchorage to the back teeth, as the device worked to tip the forward teeth toward the back. By doing this, it was felt that the teeth could move faster and without pulling the back teeth forward.

The development of the Dr. Andrews's Straight-Wire Appliance, however, caused the Tip-Edge to fall out of favor, although some orthodontists still use it today. The Tip-Edge appliance was mainly designed to help treat four-bicuspid extraction cases (which accounted for 60–70 percent of all cases during the 1970s and 1980s). Yet, as more cases are treated with nonextraction, these appliances fell out of favor and are not used that much anymore.

LINGUAL

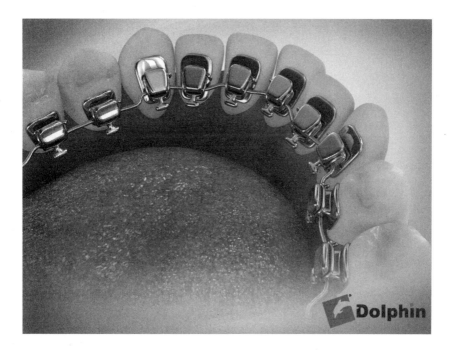

Lingual braces are similar to the braces most of us are familiar with, except that they were developed to be placed on the tongue side, instead of the lip side, of the teeth. They were mainly developed in response to the aesthetic demands of patients, especially older teens and adults who wanted straight teeth without showing their braces. Patients who want orthodontic treatment but don't want their appliances to be obvious will sometimes opt for lingual braces. Prior to Invisalign, lingual braces were the only aesthetic option for orthodontic treatment. Although there were clear braces and tooth-colored wires, they were still somewhat noticeable and not invisible.

Lingual braces work in the same manner as standard braces: by holding a wire in a slot, thus delivering continuous pressure to the teeth in a certain direction. However, while the length of treatment time with lingual braces should theoretically be the same as it is with standard braces, the reality is that most lingual cases take slightly longer to finish. The mechanics used to move the teeth are similar to that of traditional braces, but there is much less research and training with these appliances.

Today, lingual braces—like many other braces on the market—can be customized and placed with computer-determined, ideal placement of the brackets, which helps increase efficiency and decrease time of the treatment. Popular brands include Incognito, iBraces, In-Ovation, and SureSmile Lingual.

It's important to keep in mind, however, that because these lingual braces are custom-made, the lab fees can run high, which adds to the cost. Typically, lingual braces can cost anywhere from 25 to 100 percent more than traditional braces. Additionally, the interior placement of the braces can become bothersome to the tongue and can affect chewing, swallowing, and speech. In addition, breakage problems are more common with lingual braces than with traditional braces.

SELF-LIGATING BRACES

There are three main parts to braces: the brace, which is cemented onto the tooth; the wire, which is inserted into the slot of braces and delivers a constant force to move the teeth; and the elastomeric ties, which hold the wire in the slot of the braces. While effective in their own right, traditional braces have some inefficiencies that have been addressed through a series of evolutions over the years.

For example, many orthodontists realized when teeth slid along the arch wire, the elastomeric ties would create friction that would slightly impede the speed of movement. This led to the development of SPEED Braces in the 1980s, which used a metal clip instead of the troublesome elastomeric tie to hold the wire in the bracket slot. These were the first self-ligating (self-tying-off) braces. When practitioners began using this device, they noticed that the initial movement of the teeth was faster and quicker and that the teeth tended to align a little faster.

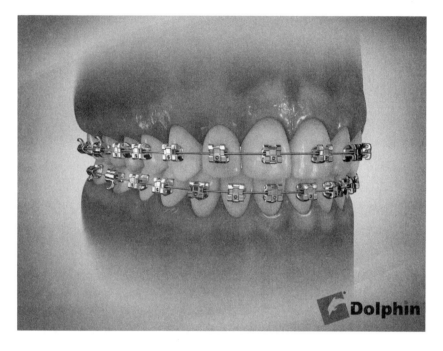

Self-ligating brackets. Notice there are no elastic ligature to hold in the arch wire.

After the development of SPEED Braces, other self-ligating devices emerged, including the Damon bracket, which used lighter arch wires and less force to achieve the same results; it was able to accomplish this due to less friction in the brackets. With less pressure placed on the teeth, there was less restriction of blood flow, which theoretically allowed for more and faster tooth movement and, ultimately, a shorter time in braces for the patient. The teeth were allowed to move in concert with the biology of the tissues.

In my experience with self-ligating braces, I've noticed that the initial alignment of the teeth does happen faster—but that is only part of the treatment. In the final phases of treatment, you need to be able to add small details in order to finish the case to ideal. Remember, most braces are not customized for each patient. Braces are designed to an average. It's the orthodontist's job to adapt the appliances to each and every patient. These devices may speed up the process at the beginning, but overall, they end up taking about as long to complete treatment as traditional braces.

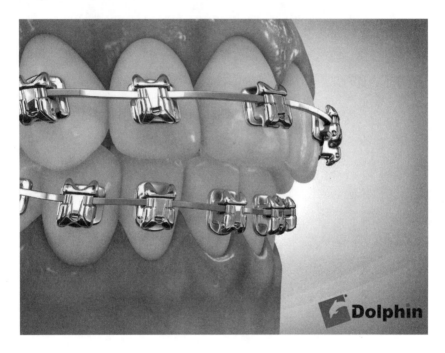

While it is true that using lighter forces helps the teeth move faster, lighter forces can be applied with any brace, not just self-ligating braces. The wire creates the force. The size and type of wire determines the force levels applied. However, it is not true that the lighter forces of self-ligating braces can encourage the growth of more bone. Some erroneously believe that, as teeth move outward toward the edge of the bone, more bone will be made to support the teeth in their new position—but this has never proven to be the case. In fact, Dr. Enlow, one of the leaders in the field of oral growth and development, has shown that moving teeth outward toward the cheek (i.e., toward the *buccal surface* of the jaw) will not cause more bone to grow in this area.[18] If teeth are moved too far out of the support tissue, the bone and gingiva will start to thin and eventually recede.

REMOVABLE FUNCTIONAL ORTHODONTIC APPLIANCES

Removable functional orthodontic devices are also popular and are active in moving the jaws and teeth. These devices, as with the ones we've discussed earlier, have evolved significantly over the years, and some have proven so effective that they are still in use today. There are hundreds of different types of removable appliances. However, here are several of the more well-known, removable functional orthodontic appliances:

- the Monobloc, developed by Dr. Robin in 1902

- the Activator, developed by Dr. Anderson in 1908

- the Bionator, developed by Dr. Balters in the 1960s

- the Frankel appliance, developed by Dr. Rolf Frankel in 1967

- the Twin Block appliance, developed by Dr. Clark in 1977

---

18 Self Edin, et al., "Do Self Ligating Bracket systems produce actual Alveolar Bone Expansion?," *IOSR Journal of Dental and Medical Sciences* 14, no. 8 (August 2015): 45-53, https://doi.org/10.9790/0853-14824553.

THE ACTIVATOR

While the Monobloc was never widely adopted, the Activator was one of the first widely used functional appliances created to correct the function of the jaws. It was mainly used throughout Europe, but was also used in the American orthodontic community throughout the 1960s and 1970s.

The mode of action for the Activator involved Anderson's theory that isometric muscular contraction was caused by myotatic reflex activity. In other words, he thought that by helping control the muscles and tissues around the teeth and helping to reposition the jaws, you could help control the alignment of the teeth and correct the bite at the same time.

However, the biggest problem with the Activator was that it was incredibly bulky and difficult both to place in the mouth and to wear; it was also almost impossible to speak with. Additionally, even though it was a removable device, it had to be worn twenty-four hours a day to be most effective.

THE BIONATOR

The Bionator, developed in the 1960s, was an improvement on the Activator in that it allowed more room for the tongue, so patients could actually speak while wearing it. The developer of the Bionator, Dr. Balters, believed that the tongue was the center reflex in the oral cavity and that the abnormal activity of that muscle could lead to the deformation of the dental arches and of lower jaw growth. By creating this appliance to reposition both the jaws and the tongue, his idea was to create equilibrium between the tongue, the muscles around the mouth, and the teeth, so they would all work in harmony.

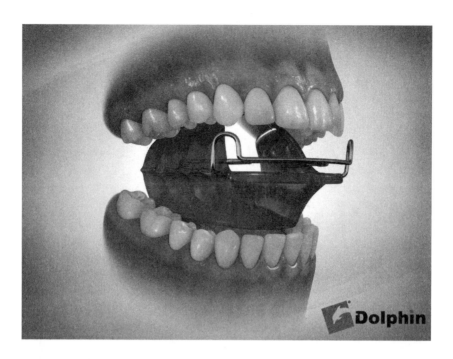

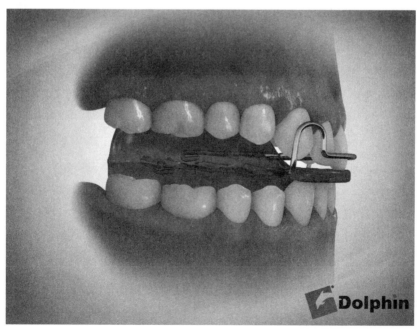

The Bionator appliance.

THE FRANKEL APPLIANCE

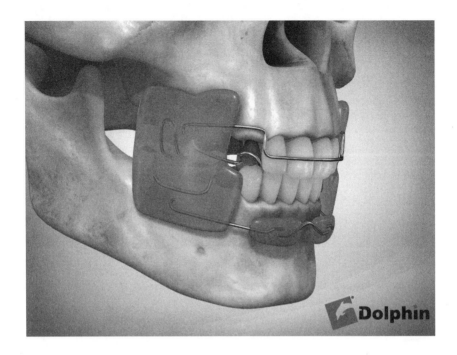

The Frankel appliance, also based on the Activator, was created by Dr. Rolf Frankel in East Germany in 1967 in response to the mixed results achieved by the Bionator variation.

Holding a slightly different view than that of Dr. Balters, Dr. Frankel believed that a treatment outcome was more stable if the functional deviations of the muscles were corrected at the same time as the teeth. The Frankel appliance was created to reprogram the muscles around the mouth to enhance favorable growth in the developing dentition. This was done by restricting undesirable muscle forces from pushing the jaws and teeth into bad positions and by encouraging the teeth and jaws to naturally move into an ideal position and relationship.

Dr. Frankel eventually developed more appliances based on this concept, including devices to address issues like Class 3 malocclusions (bad bites), open bites, bimaxillary protrusion (the tendency of the jaws to protrude outward and the front teeth to tip outward), vertical maxillary excess (where the gums on the upper jaw show excessively when smiling), and other common malocclusions.

Despite these advances, all of these devices—the Activator, the Bionator, and the Frankel—were notoriously difficult to wear and fell out of favor as new appliances that were easier to wear, were cemented to the teeth, and achieved similar results were introduced to the market.

TWIN BLOCK

Developed in 1977, the Twin Block device was created by Dr. Clark as an evolution of the Activator and Activator-like appliances mentioned earlier. It consisted of two retainers with blocks placed where the teeth from both jaws touched (the occlusal portion) so that the jaw moved into an ideal position every time the patient bit down. It's mainly used to correct a Class 2 jaw relationship, where the lower jaw is too far back from the upper jaw.

As with the Activator and associated appliances, the philosophy behind the Twin Block is that in encouraging the patient to function in this position—with the jaw moving more forward into an ideal Class 1 position—the musculature and jaws would develop to take an ideal position on their own.

What doctors found with the Twin Block was that the device helped reposition the lower jaw and caused the back teeth to intrude (to move slightly downward, into the jaw bone, thus "shortening" them). By intruding the posterior teeth, the lower jaw has to rotate more to close. It is this "auto rotation" of the lower jaw that helps bring it more forward and into a better alignment with the upper jaw.

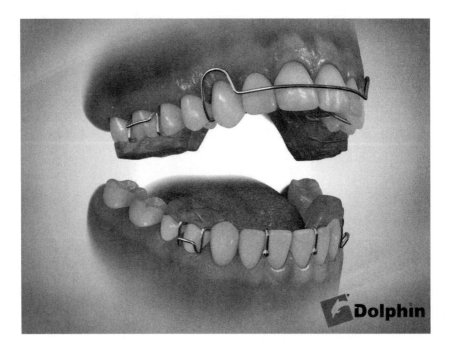

In other words, the jaws will naturally close until the teeth touch, so by bringing the posterior (back) teeth of the upper jaw back, the lower jaw will naturally move up and forward to complete that bite.

Just as with the Activator-like appliances, the Twin Block—though removable—should be worn twenty-four hours a day in order to be fully effective. The Twin Block isn't as difficult to wear as its predecessors, although it's still somewhat bulky and is separated into two pieces instead of one, with one fitted on the upper jaw and one on the lower. This makes inserting the device a little easier as well, and while speaking and eating can still be somewhat challenging, they are still easier to do than with the earlier devices.

SPRING RETAINERS

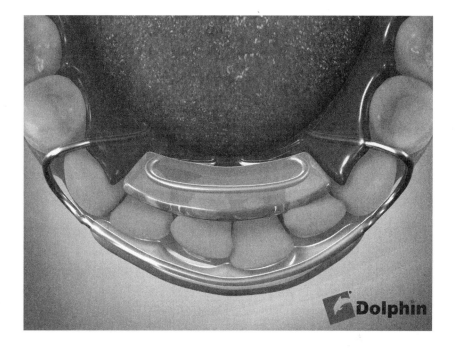

Another simpler, removable device that is not based on the Activator is the spring retainer. It is essentially a retainer with small springs inserted, each of which is designed to move an individual tooth or a group of teeth. While this device doesn't move the teeth at their base, it does create a tipping force on the tooth, helping to bring slightly off-center or canted teeth into alignment. This appliance does not correct the jaw relationship, but is focused on minor movements of a few specific teeth or groups of teeth.

Adjunct Appliances

ELASTICS

Elastics are the small rubber bands of varying sizes and strengths that hook onto appliances and help move them in a certain direction.

Although about 90 percent of movement with elastics is dental movement—making them more of an orthodontic appliance rather than orthopedic—there is a small component of skeletal movement achieved with elastics.

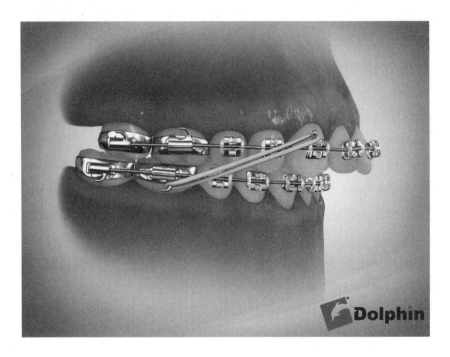

Alternative Appliances

CLEAR ALIGNERS

Clear aligners, one of the most common of which is Invisalign, are basically an adaptation from clear retainers. A series of clear retainers are used to progressively move the teeth until they're in an ideal bite. The Invisalign system uses digital computer-aided design and manufacturing (CAD/CAM) technology to help the orthodontist achieve that ideal bite, all of which I address more in the next chapter.

Regardless of which removable functional appliance is worn, most orthodontists will recommend that treatment last a minimum of nine months to maximum of eighteen months, depending on the severity of the bad bite, how fast the patient is growing, and how often the patient wears the device.

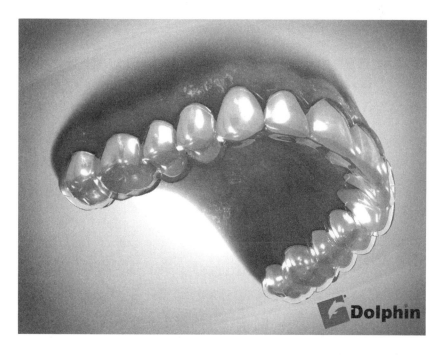

Chapter 5 Summary

- There are two types of appliances used in orthodontics: orthodontic and orthopedic. Orthodontic devices are used to correct the teeth, while orthopedic devices modify the growth of the bones.

- Orthodontic devices deliver lighter, constant forces over time, while orthopedic devices are often heavier and apply more pressure in order to effect both skeletal and dental movement.

- Edgewise appliances, invented by Dr. Edward Angle in the 1920s, are the forerunner of today's modern braces.

- Advances in braces, such as lingual braces and the ability to bond brackets directly to the teeth, have led to more effective and less visible braces.

- Orthopedic devices may be used to widen the upper jaw or to shift the jaw's position to bring it into a more ideal bite position.

- Apart from the use of orthopedic devices, skeletal discrepancies can also be treated with dental camouflage, orthognathic surgery, or growth modification.

- Common orthopedic devices include palatal expanders, headgear, protraction facemasks, and chin cup appliances.

- Fixed functional orthopedic appliances are cemented to the teeth in order to effect jaw growth and were created in response to the need for appliances that were easier to wear for patients who had a hard time complying with removable devices. These appliances include the Herbst and MARA devices.

- Orthodontic devices put pressure on the teeth and can be either fixed or removable.

- Braces are the most common fixed orthodontic appliance, and come in three main types: Edgewise appliances of varying prescriptions, lingual, and self-ligating.

- Removable orthodontic appliances include the Twin Block appliance, spring retainers, and clear aligners.

Invisalign

nvisalign technology—the clear-aligner alternative to braces—was invented in 1997 by Stanford business students Zia Chishti and Kelsey Wirth.

The idea began with Chishti, a former orthodontic patient who hadn't worn his retainer as a teenager and later found that his teeth had shifted. What Chishti didn't know, and what a lot of people don't realize, is that your teeth will shift your entire life, even into your eighties.

It wasn't until college that Chishti finally went to an orthodontist, who recommended he get braces to correct the drift and straighten his teeth. Chishti was against the idea, likely because of a perceived stigma around braces on adults, and asked if there were any alternatives. The only option his orthodontist could offer him was something called an Essix retainer.

Essix retainer technology is an approach to teeth alignment that has been around since the early 1980s. It involves a vacuum-formed removable retainer made from clear material such as polypropylene or polyvinylchloride that is almost invisible against the teeth. To make the retainer, a mold is taken of the teeth, and the plastic is formed around the model. The resulting retainer can either be used to hold the teeth in place or to move the teeth incrementally, carefully removing the molds of the individual teeth from the mold of the jaw and moving them in set intervals, creating new molds from the new positions to gradually pressure the teeth into an improved alignment.

Patients using the Essix retainer to move their teeth need to wear it for several weeks in each stage, often using several trays to move the teeth into abetter position.

Chishti's thought was that if you could do this process manually, by taking a mold of the teeth and physically moving the teeth within the model, then the same technology could be applied with computers. Using CAD/CAM technology, the patient's teeth could be recreated in a virtual 3D environment, and 3D models could be printed out for each stage of tooth movement, instead of handcrafting each step.

That concept was the beginning of Invisalign.

THE BONES BEHIND INVISALIGN

Toward the end of 1997, Invisalign began testing its new product on volunteer patients, starting with clinical tests at the University of the Pacific's orthodontic program, where I was fortunate to be a student.

Although the appliance wasn't even close to what it is today, I remember being impressed by the concept. In fact, the orthodontists who worked on those early Invisalign cases at UOP were also able to develop a best-practices protocol in 2007 so that other professionals could learn from their discoveries over the years and have the most success.

As with the Essix retainer, the appliance is based on the fact that constant force on a tooth will result in the tooth's movement. It doesn't matter if that force is applied by braces, an aligner, a retainer, or by the tongue, cheek, or lips. The tooth will respond by moving if the force is constant enough.

The reason for this is just one of the amazing aspects of the human body: the constant rebuilding of living bone. In life, our bones are not static structures. As the main source of calcium for our bodies, our bones are the first place our body goes to restore this mineral, resorbing bone mass and sending it into the bloodstream. On the other hand, if the body doesn't need the calcium, it replaces the mineral back into the bone. These actions are performed by bone cells called osteoclasts (bone absorbers) and osteoblasts (bone builders).

Thanks to bone cells, when you put force on a tooth, osteoclasts eat away at the bone in front of the force, allowing the tooth and its root to move. Behind the movement, the osteoblasts lay down more bone to fill in the gap. Depending on the direction of the force, the tooth can move in three dimensions—in or out, up or down, and left or right. In fact, the movement of the tooth is really only limited by the small connective tissue that attaches the root of the tooth to the bone: the periodontal ligament. Apart from that limitation, it's up to the appliance to put the most accurate direction of force on the tooth to get it to move in the desired direction.

EVOLUTION OF INVISALIGN

Since Invisalign was released in 1997, its percentage of effective treatments has improved dramatically: from about 5 percent of all cases when it first came out to around 80 percent as of 2016. The reason for this is the organization's development of tooth movement technologies, which have improved year after year—in some cases, dramatically. Following is a brief breakdown of the advancements Invisalign has made over the course of fifteen years:

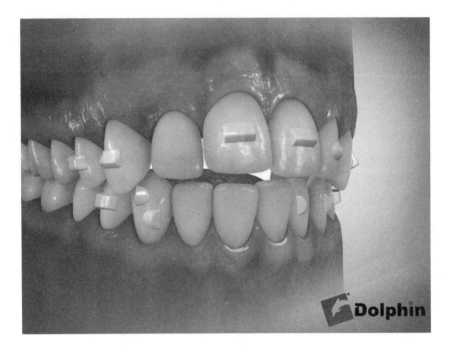

- **2002**: Tooth-colored composite bumps are developed that can be glued onto the teeth, changing the surface so that the aligner can engage more with the tooth and encourage it in a certain direction.

- **2002–2009**: SmartForce Clinical Innovations are invented, and multiple generations are released over the years. Innovations include precision cuts in plastic so elastics could be used in conjunction with the trays, as well as power ridges, which apply torque to the tooth, allowing both the tooth and the root to move simultaneously.

Because of these innovations, Invisalign moves from only being able to treat Class 1 bites, which are fairly good bites, to treating Class 2 and 3 bites, which were formerly relegated to braces-only treatment.

- **2009**: The first wave of SmartForce optimized attachments, called *G2*, is released, allowing aligners to deliver more accurate and efficient force to the tooth and move it in a desired direction. This same year, a virtual model is created in conjunction with a physical apparatus to measure force levels and torque. Combined, these models allow for better tracking of the appliance's effectiveness.

- **2010**: SmartForceG3 is released, which includes an optimized rotation attachment, optimized extrusion attachments, and refined power ridges for torque control. The rotation and extrusion movements had been very difficult for Invisalign to accomplish before these attachments were developed, often driving orthodontists to use other means to affect these movements. With the new attachments, orthodontists were able to make those movements within the Invisalign appliance, which improved the efficiency and predictability of the results across the board.

MORE CONSTANT FORCE TO IMPROVE CONTROL OF TOOTH MOVEMENTS

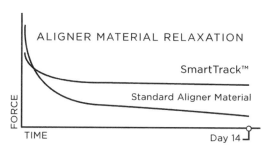

ALIGNER MATERIAL RELAXATION

SmartTrack™

Standard Aligner Material

FORCE

TIME

Day 14

- **2011**: SmartForce G4 is released, which includes new attachments for better root movement control, as well as a significant change to the material used in making Invisalign trays. After eight years of research and development, Align introduces a new aligner material. The properties of the new material, called **SmartTrack**, parallel the properties of a super-elastic, nickel-titanium wire, which allows for a lower initial force level on the teeth that stays constant over time. The material is more elastic than previously used aligner material. The elasticity also allows the material to form over very crooked teeth while still being easy to remove and makes the tray more comfortable to wear. Lastly, the material allows for greater flexibility in the use of attachments, allowing orthodontists to use more attachments comfortably, without having to choose some and leave others off for the sake of patient comfort. This same year, a multi-tooth movement approach is released that allows separate movements for separate sections of the mouth, making it possible for conditions such as open bites to be treated with Invisalign.

- **2012**: The SmartForce G5 release includes new mechanics to treat deep overbites, which were difficult for Invisalign to accomplish before the technology was created to move separate sets of teeth in different directions. With this release, the movements needed to correct overbites become much more accurate. Additionally, optimized extrusion attachments for the bicuspids that also assist with overbite correction are created, as well as Bite Turbos, which function as a small ledge cemented onto the tooth that assists with tooth movement. It was these "deep bite" mechanics that improved the device all-around and allowed for treatment of more serious Class 2 and Class 3 bites with more accurate and predictable results.

- **2015**: The SmartForceG6 release brings a lot of the previous advancements together to develop better closure of tooth extraction sites, a process that formerly could only be achieved with braces. This release also includes optimized anchorage and retraction attachments, as well as SmartStage technology, which allows for more accurate and controlled movements of specific teeth to close up extraction sites, opening up another 20 percent of the patient population that could be helped with Invisalign.

- **2016**: Instead of new attachments, the SmartForceG7 release decreases the time a patient uses each progressing retainer from an average of fourteen days to seven, speeding up the treatment process as a whole.

Because of these advancements, more orthodontists understand the value of Invisalign and see it as more than just a plastic tray with movement built in. Instead, the system is now a refined approach to tooth movement that allows for very specific force in focused and multiple directions to achieve predictable movements with accurate results.

THE INVISALIGN PROCESS

A typical Invisalign treatment begins with a scan of the teeth to create a three-dimensional model that's accurate down to fifty microns, or about the width of a human hair. The scan is used to create a 3D model in the Invisalign software, which the orthodontist then manipulates to create a virtual plan of how the teeth should move to be brought into alignment. The software then designs the clear aligners needed for these movements to take place, and the trays are manufactured all at once, from the beginning to the end of the treatment.

About every seven days, the patient is given a new tray to wear, and each tray must be worn a minimum of twenty-two hours every day. This extended wear time is important, as it's the consistency of the force that causes the tooth to move. If the aligner is worn for less time, it loses effectiveness. In total, Invisalign treatments typically take around twenty months to complete, and the resulting movement of the teeth is similar to what you'd see with braces.

BRACES VERSUS INVISALIGN

The main difference between braces and Invisalign is the force directed to a tooth is more of a pulling mechanism with braces, while there is a pushing force with Invisalign. However, a tooth doesn't really care what direction the force is coming from; it just responds to that force by moving away from it.

When it comes to choosing braces or Invisalign, there are three main factors to consider:

1. Is the patient diligent enough to wear the tray twenty-two hours a day? Invisalign is easy to remove, but it's also easy to forget to put it back in. If the tray is left out for several hours, multiple days in a row, the treatment won't be very effective. Remember, orthodontic movement requires a constant force. Once the force is removed, the teeth will slowly move back toward the previous position.

2. How complex is the case? There are some movements that are difficult, if not impossible, for Invisalign to achieve,

though that gap is closing (no pun intended) with each new iteration of the system.

3. Lastly, there's the orthodontist's knowledge of how to move the teeth with Invisalign. If a dentist or orthodontist doesn't understand how the teeth move with Invisalign and tries to create a movement that's either difficult or impossible to do with the aligners, then the treatment may not only fail—it may make the teeth worse.

Just like with braces, the use of Invisalign requires a lot of training, not only in understanding how to move the teeth but also in practical, hands-on experience and an in the overarching understanding of the biomechanics and physiology of tooth movement.

CASE STUDY: INVISALIGN VERSUS JAW SURGERY

In 2014, a patient of mine asked what I could do about a fairly significant anterior open bite (where none of the front teeth touch when biting down) she was suffering from. She'd seen six other orthodontists before me, and each of them recommended jaw surgery. At sixty-seven years old, however, she hesitated undergo something so dramatic and invasive, because she was worried about the recovery time and the risks associated with surgery.

But her bite was a serious problem. For years, she'd only been able to chew with her very back teeth—none of her other teeth touched. And because she couldn't chew well, it affected her diet and, consequently, her health. She suffered from headaches and overall had a very poor quality of life. She told me she wanted to correct her bite so she could "chew a sandwich."

Fortunately, Invisalign is great at intruding teeth down into the bone, especially in the back of the mouth, which was where she needed the most movement. By intruding the posterior teeth, the lower jaw can auto rotate and close down in the anterior. Not only does this close the open bite in the anterior, but it also helps correct the Class 2 overjet. By intruding the posterior teeth and bringing the front teeth to a position where they contacted the opposing arch, we could at least get her close to a normal function.

I told her about her options—either jaw surgery or the possibilities with Invisalign—and she decided to give Invisalign a try first.

After twenty-two months of treatment, we were able to achieve excellent results, bringing her jaw into an ideal bite without even a hint of surgery. She had her first salad in years, as well as that sandwich she'd wanted for so long. And because she was finally able to eat healthier food, she ended up losing twenty-five pounds over the next year. It was an incredible result and a relief to the patient knowing that she wouldn't have to undergo the trauma of surgery.

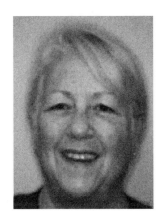

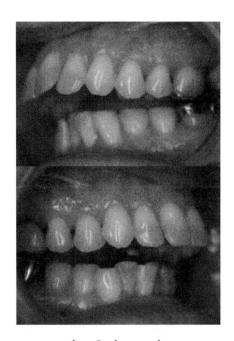

BEFORE: Patient with an anterior open bite. In the past, this would have been treated almost exclusively with surgery.

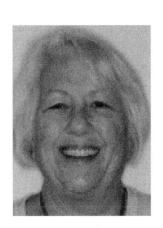

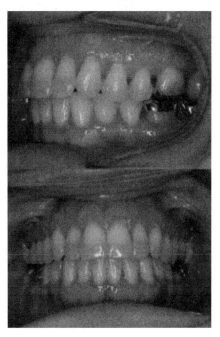

AFTER: Patient after twenty-two months of Invisalign treatments. No surgery was needed.

COMMON MYTHS ABOUT INVISALIGN

There are two big myths out there about Invisalign: (1) it doesn't work or (2) it works for all cases.

The reason for the first myth lies in the early success rate of the system. When Invisalign first came out, its success rate was around 5 percent. Every few years, however, the system has improved in accuracy, effectiveness, and efficiency, leading to its current success rate.

To answer the latter myth, as long as it's used correctly, Invisalign will work for about 80 percent of orthodontic cases. As for the remaining 20 percent, the system still has a difficult time accomplishing certain movements, such as moving molars a long distance (more than 5–6mm), a task for which braces are currently better suited. This is because of the natural tipping action of the tooth as it moves. When traversing longer distances within the mouth, a tooth will tip to one side, upright itself, then tip again, over and over until it comes to rest. With braces, the wire keeps the tooth upright and moving bodily in the correct direction. With Invisalign, there is no wire to keep the tooth upright, leaving the tooth to tip if it moves too far. Although Align Technology is aware of this and has developed force mechanisms within the aligner to help keep the tooth upright, the technology mainly works for the canine and bicuspids. However, it's likely only a matter of time before Invisalign develops an appliance that controls this tipping over longer distances.

Chapter 6 Summary

- Align Technology, Inc., the innovators of Invisalign—the clear-aligner alternative to braces—was founded in 1997 by two Stanford business students: Zia Chishti and Kelsey Wirth.

- Invisalign technology is based on the Essix retainer, which is a plastic mold around a model of the teeth, in which the teeth have been adjusted slightly so that the wearer's teeth are moved by incremental steps into their ideal position. Invisalign took this concept a step further by using CAD/CAM technology and software to more accurately determine the best movement of the teeth and to create the progression of retainers needed to bring the teeth into an ideal bite.

- A scan of the teeth is done to create a 3D model, which the orthodontist then manipulates to create a virtual model of how the teeth should move in order to bring them into alignment. The software then designs the aligners needed for these movements to take place, and all of the trays are manufactured at once.

- Invisalign trays are switched out every seven days or less, and each tray must be worn a minimum of twenty-two hours a day. If it's worn less, the treatment won't be as effective.

- The main difference between braces and Invisalign, apart from appearance, is that braces use a pulling force to move teeth, while Invisalign uses a pushing force.

- Invisalign requires extensive training to implement correctly, so be sure your orthodontist has an in-depth understanding of how Invisalign works, as well as practical, hands-on experience.

- When done correctly, Invisalign works for about 80 percent of orthodontic cases.

Accelerated and Surgical Orthodontics

O ne of the biggest complaints and challenges about orthodontic treatment is the length of time it takes to complete
treatment. The average duration of orthodontic treatment
is nineteen months to two years. There are many patients that would
love to have their teeth straightened and bites corrected, but do not
want to endure two years of braces or aligners. In addition, the longer
the treatment times the more risks patients take on. Risks such as
caries (cavities), white spot lesions, and root resorption, all increase
with time in treatment. Moreover, longer treatment times lead to
lower patient satisfaction rates and less compliance with treatments.
Thus, methods and techniques to reduce treatment time can not only
reduce the risks associated with lengthy orthodontic treatment, but

also help aid in patient compliance and patient satisfaction with the results.

Accelerated orthodontics, however, is not a one-step process. There are several factors involved that will affect treatment time, and each one is unique to every patient:

1. The complexity of the case

2. Amount of tooth movement required

3. Amount of skeletal change required

4. The patient's biological response to the orthodontic forces applied

5. The amount of patient cooperation required

In addition, the experience and expertise of each orthodontist also plays a big factor in the speed of treatment.

A PROPER DIAGNOSIS AND THE ABILITY TO CREATE AN EFFICIENT, EFFECTIVE TREATMENT PLAN

An orthodontist will study the case and all of its complexities to create an ideal treatment plan, allowing for all orthodontic corrections needed and how those corrections can be made in a minimal amount of time.

A THOROUGH UNDERSTANDING OF ORTHODONTIC BIOMECHANICS

An orthodontist must select the appropriate movements and appliances that will create the movement needed to form an ideal bite in the most efficient manner possible. If the treatment involves a lot of patient cooperation and compliance, and the patient either has, or admits to having, a history of poor compliance, the orthodontist may need to consider using a self-activating appliance or one that takes the factor of patient cooperation out of the picture.

ADVANCES IN THE UNDERSTANDING OF TOOTH MOVEMENT

Since the founding of orthodontics at the beginning of the nineteenth century, orthodontists have assumed that a person's biology was individualized and unchangeable.

Accelerating orthodontic treatment has always been on the minds of orthodontists and their patients, but only in the last twenty to thirty years has there been any significant advances in this area. Many researchers have tried to improve the mechanics of tooth movement through the use of

- computer-generated custom arch wires,

- body-heat activated arch wires,

- self-ligating brackets,

- computer-aided indirect bonding, and

- improved bracket prescriptions and design.

Some of these have been shown to have improved treatment efficiency, but not necessarily shorten treatment time. There are fewer visits and adjustments required in order to finish treatment. However, in order to decrease treatment time researchers have been focused on speeding up the rate of tooth movement at the biological level. In order for teeth to move through the bone, the bone cells called osteoclasts, need to break down the bone in front of the movement, and bone cells called osteoblasts behind the movement need to form new bone to fill in the area from where the tooth has moved. Numerous studies have been done to document the cellular markers that help initiate this bone metabolism. Using this information, scientists have tried to discover triggers that can not only help initiate this reaction, but also increase and magnify the reaction in order to speed up the cellular processes associated with bone metabolism and thus, tooth movement. Some of these include:

- Pulsed electromagnetic fields

- Lower level mechanical vibration

- Low-level laser therapy

- Corticocision

- Decortication of the bone

- Piezocision

- Micro-osteoperforation

- Piezoelectricity

- Injection of pharmacological agents such as:

  □ Prostaglandins

  □ Relaxins

  □ Platelet-rich plasma

Most of these have had little effectiveness in speeding up or accelerating tooth movement. The ones that show the most promise but need further study are decortication of the bone, corticocision, piezocision, micro-osteoperforation, and low-level laser therapy.

DISCOVERY OF ACCELERATED TOOTH MOVEMENT METHODS

Dentists and orthodontists have known for a long time that tooth movement varies depending on the type of bone that the teeth are moving through. For instance, teeth in *trabecular bone*—bone that appears spongier and less dense—move at a faster rate than teeth in cortical, or denser, bone. Because of this difference, they believe the density of the bone plays an important part in the rate of movement, and if the density of the bone is reduced, the overall rate of movement would increase. Additionally, an increase in inflammatory markers in the bone, like those which occurs after the bone has been injured in some way, has been associated with a rate of tooth movement 2.3 times faster than the average rate.[19]

Based on these theories, surgeons have been using *corticotomy* procedures—a series of cuts into the bone around the teeth—to increase the rate of tooth movement since the 1950s.

CORTICOTOMY FACILITATED TOOTH MOVEMENT

Several authors have described accelerated tooth movement in conjunction with corticotomy procedures. In 1959, Kole reported that combining a corticotomy surgery with orthodontic treatment he was able to complete cases of active orthodontic tooth movements within twelve weeks. The surgery consisted of laying a gingival flap and exposing the bone tissue surrounding the teeth. Cuts were made

---

19   Teixeira, C, et al., "Cytokine Expression and Accelerated Tooth Movement," Journal of Dental Research 89, no. 10 (2010): 1135–1141, https://doi. org/10.1177/0022034510373764; Alikhani, Mani et al., "Effect of micro-osteo-perforations on the rate of tooth movement," American Journal of Orthodontics and Dentofacial Orthopedics 144, no. 4, 639–648.

through the dense cortical bone into the less dense medullary and trabecular bone. Other researchers like Suya in 1991 treated 394 patients with corticotomy surgeries and finished all of the orthodontic cases within twelve months. He also reported that much of the orthodontic movement was finished within the first three months following the corticotomy procedures. Many other orthodontists were able to reproduce similar results following corticotomy procedures. This phenomenon was termed "Regional Acceleratory Phenomenon" by orthopedist Harold Frost in 1989 when describing the healing process that occurs when bones are cut during surgical procedures. He collectively termed this cascade of physiologic healing events the regional acceleratory phenomenon (RAP). RAP healing is a complex physiologic process with dominating features involving accelerated bone turnover and decreases in regional bone densities.[20]

DECORTICATION OF THE BONE/ WILCKODONTICS

In the 1990s, the Wilcko brothers—one an orthodontist and the other a periodontist—took these corticotomy procedures a step further when they found that some of their patients who required bone grafting before having braces put in were having much quicker results in tooth movement than other patients. After studying those cases, the Wilcko brothers concluded that this increased movement occurred because the cuts in the bone around the teeth caused the bone's mineralization process to slow down, allowing the teeth to

---

20   Köle H., "Surgical operations of the alveolar ridge to correct occlusal abnormalities," *Oral Surg Oral Med Oral Pathol* 12, (1959): 515–529; Suya H., *Mechanical and Biological Basics in Orthodontic Therapy* (Heidelberg: Hütlig Buch, 1991), 207–226; Frost HM, "The biology of fracture healing: An overview for clinicians. Part I," *Clin Orthop Rel Res* 248 (1989):283–293.

move faster. This discovery led the brothers, in 2001, to patent the procedures as Accelerated Osteogenic Orthodontic technique (AOO), which soon became known by orthodontists as *Wilckodontics*.[21]

DECORTICATION/WILCKODONTICS PROCEDURE

The Wilckodontics procedure involves folding back a full thickness of gum tissue to expose the bone around the teeth, also known as the *alveolar bone*. Once the alveolar bone is exposed, it's scored and perforated along the roots of the teeth, and the scored area of bone is removed and replaced with a freeze-dried bone graft.

As a result, the bone goes through a two-month healing phase known as *osteopenia*, where the mineral content of the bone significantly decreases, allowing the teeth to move within the bone at 50–75 percent faster than the normal rate.

However, even though the Wilckodontic corticotomy procedure is very effective, there is a fair amount of post-surgical discomfort; sutures are usually involved, and there are typically several follow-up visits. Additionally, heavy pain medications are often prescribed to help relieve pain during the two-week recovery period, which may keep the patient out of work and off the road for a longer period of time.

MICRO-OSTEOPERFORATION

Micro-osteoperforation is another accelerated tooth movement procedure based on the theory that bone that is in the process of

---

21   Wilcko WM, et al., "Rapid orthodontics with alveolar reshaping: two case reports of decrowding," *Int J Periodontics Restorative Dent* 21, (2001): 9-19.

healing allows for a significantly improved rate of tooth movement. However, instead of grafting new bone in, the process relies on the bone's reaction to injury.

When our bones are injured, they activate a repair mechanism that removes the injured bone and builds new bone—a process called *osteoclastic activity*. During this short period of healing time, inflammatory markers called *cytokines* and *chemokines* increase their bone-absorbing activity, reducing the bone density near the injured area and allowing the teeth to move more quickly while the bone is healing.

THE MICRO-OSTEOPERFORATION PROCESS

In practice, micro-osteoperforation involves making a series of very fine holes in the alveolar bone, as close as possible to the teeth that must be moved. As the bone reacts to the small injury, the nearby teeth are able to move 50–75 percent faster than average during the healing process. This process can last from eight to sixteen weeks.

To create these micro-perforations, the NYU Department of Orthodontics developed a device called the Propel, which looks like a thick marker with a small screw about the size of a ballpoint pen tip on the end.

EVOLUTION OF THE PROPEL DEVICE

When the Propel device was first released by the NYU Department of Orthodontics in 2012, it was designed as a single-use, sterile, disposable, and manual perforator with a metal tip equipped with a depth collar to indicate how deep the screw was inserted.

The second-generation Propel improved on the first with a sturdier structure composed mainly of metal, which allowed for more leverage and balance when inserting the screw. In this second generation, the handle could be removed for sterilization purposes, and the screw was disposable.

For generation three, the device was redesigned with a disposable screw tip and automatic torque driver so that the orthodontist didn't have to manually turn the screw into the bone—a process that presented a challenge when it came to the thicker cortical bone.

Due to the advances in the Propel device, micro-osteoperforation is quickly becoming one of the most promising procedures for increasing the rate of tooth movement in adult patients.

During the procedure, the gum area is numbed with a topical jelly anesthesia; a local anesthetic is often injected as well. Once numbed, the orthodontist uses the Propel device to screw into the bone to the proper depth (between 3 mm and 7 mm) and then removes the screw from the tissue. This process is repeated about two or three times for each tooth, as the inflammation response needed will only occur within 5–6 mm of the perforation. If the whole mouth is being done, up to sixty perforations may be made. There may be some minor bleeding as a result of the procedure, but this is often a very small amount that stops entirely within fifteen minutes. There may also be some mild to moderate discomfort to the gums for the twenty-four to thirty-six hours following the procedure, but this can be minimized with over-the-counter Tylenol (acetaminophen).

The candidates who benefit the most from this procedure are typically adults who are no longer growing, as they lack the growth hormone in the body that tends to naturally speed up tooth movement. Additionally, the patient should only opt to undergo the osteoperforation process if it will result in a significant improvement on the length of an orthodontic procedure. For instance, if an adult patient has a simple case that can be completed in six to seven months, the osteoperforation procedure would only take an extra one or two months off the total time—a difference that is likely not worth the extra effort.

However, if the patient is an adult and the case is fairly complex—possibly requiring about eighteen months to finish—then the osteoperforation process could reduce that time by about 40 percent, completing the case in about ten to eleven months instead of eighteen. A twenty-four-month case could be completed in thirteen to fourteen months, and a thirty-six-month case could be done in as little as nineteen or twenty months.

Along with complex cases, osteoperforation has also been used to help with difficult and challenging movements, and to help move teeth that haven't responded well (or at all) to more standard orthodontic treatments, such as braces.

In the past few years, micro-osteoperforation has quickly become a top choice for increasing tooth movement thanks to its minimally invasive approach and efficacy in stimulating the patient's own biological responses to speed up the process.

LOW-LEVEL MECHANICAL VIBRATIONS

Apart from the advancements made with micro-osteoperforation, recent orthopedic research has also found some mounting evidence suggesting low-level mechanical vibrations can have a positive effect on bone metabolism by increasing the rate of bone remodeling— a practice currently in use for the intervention and prevention of osteoporosis.

While researchers are still working to understand the biological reasons behind these results, studies have shown that bones subjected to a vibrational force for certain periods of time each day can substantially improve their bone formation and the speed of that formation.

Another study done at the University of San Antonio compared patients undergoing orthodontic treatment who either did or did not use the vibrational pulsating device AcceleDent during their treatment.[22] They found those who used AcceleDent for twenty minutes each day had a 51 percent increase in tooth movement over those who used no vibrational pulsating device at all.

More recently however, there have been several studies showing low level mechanical vibration does not significantly increase the rate of tooth movement during orthodontics.[23]

ACCELEDENT

AcceleDent is the most common appliance used today to accelerate tooth movement. The device consists of a small, plastic bite wafer

---

22 Pavlin, Dubravko et al., "Cyclic loading (vibration) accelerates tooth movement in orthodontic patients: A double-blind, randomized controlled trial," *Seminars in Orthodontics* 21, no. 3: 187–194.

23 Leethanakul, Chidchanok, et al., "Vibratory stimulus and accelerated tooth movement: A critical appraisal," Journal of the World Federation of Orthodontists 7, no. 3: 106-112; DiBiase, Andrew T., et al., "Effects of supplemental vibrational force on space closure, treatment duration, and occlusal outcome: A multicenter randomized clinical trial," American Journal of Orthodontics and Dentofacial Orthopedics 153, no. 4: 469-480; Miles, Peter, et al., "Assessment of the rate of premolar extraction space closure in the maxillary arch with the AcceleDent Aura appliance vs no appliance in adolescents: A single-blind randomized clinical trial," American Journal of Orthodontics and Dentofacial Orthopedics 153, no. 1: 8-14.

the patient places in the target area, turning it on for an average of twenty minutes per day. During that time, the device creates a pulsating, low-magnitude, and cyclical force on the teeth and surrounding bone, accelerating the rate of bone remodeling and, in turn, increasing the rate of orthodontic tooth movement.

While this process does not have sufficient evidence to prove that it actually accelerates tooth movement, its biggest advantage is that it's noninvasive; there are no needles, no anesthesia, and no perforation of the bone.

This process does not have sufficient evidence to prove that it actually accelerates tooth movement and has other factors one should consider:

- Results can't be localized as much as with the other, more invasive procedures

- The cost can be prohibitive, with AcceleDent devices typically retailing around $1,300

- The process requires daily patient cooperation, with the patient dedicated to twenty minutes of treatment every day

MOST EFFECTIVE PROCESSES FOR ACCELERATING TOOTH MOVEMENT

After reviewing the different methods for increasing the rate of tooth movement, micro-osteoperforation and corticotomy stand out as the two most cost-effective, yet minimally invasive, procedures currently available. Micro-osteoperforation (Propel) is less invasive and less expensive than a corticotomy procedure. For patients contemplating orthodontic treatment, but hesitate because of the length of the process, these two procedures can make a significant difference, decreasing treatment times by as much as 40–50 percent while also decreasing the risks associated with orthodontic treatment, such as the following:

- susceptibility to cavities

- increased root resorption

- gingivitis

- periodontitis

- other gum and bone diseases

Although there are many factors that affect treatment time, these procedures can be the best approach to a speedy and successful overall treatment.

SURGICAL ORTHODONTICS

There are many factors that combine to create a harmonious bite, and for patients who need orthodontics treatment due to a poor bite or misaligned teeth, there's usually some component of skeletal imbalance that accompanies that poor bite. Most of these skeletal imbalances are very subtle and can either be corrected very easily during a routine orthodontic treatment or have very little—if any—impact on the bite or overall facial aesthetics.

However, the larger a skeletal discrepancy becomes, the more difficult it is to correct, to the point where orthodontic treatment alone won't be able to restore functional and aesthetic balance. Should a case become more extreme—creating a significant jaw discrepancy—orthopedic devices can be used to help modify that growth and either minimize or fully correct the skeletal imbalance, but only if the discrepancy is caught during the patient's growing years (before the late teens or early twenties).

The greatest amount of a person's face and mouth development occurs during the first fourteen to eighteen years of life, when the sutures within the skull and jaws are still forming and the use of orthopedic appliances is most effective. This is why it's vital to see an orthodontist at a young age: to catch any growth abnormalities early. If caught early enough, these abnormalities can be diagnosed and treated without having to resort to surgery. As I mentioned previously in Chapter 5, there are several options out there for modifying growth without surgery, however, many of these appliances are highly dependent on two factors: the amount of growth the patient exhibits, and the amount of time the patient wears the appliance (patient compliance).

An orthodontist has no control over either of these factors. For instance, if a patient doesn't grow at all during the course of treatment, then the appliance will have little effect. Alternately, if the patient doesn't wear the specific appliance for the respective number of hours throughout the entire treatment period, then the device will not have enough time to bring about any changes.

Another problem arises if the patient's abnormal growth pattern accelerates; even if they are fully dedicated to wearing the device according to their treatment plan, the abnormal growth may be difficult, if not impossible, to overcome.

There's also the slight chance that a patient could undergo successful orthodontic or orthopedic treatment, but once the treatment is complete, the abnormal growth pattern continues. The discrepancy can continue until it cannot be corrected with more appliances. In these cases, orthognathic (corrective jaw) surgery may be required.

WHEN ORTHOGNATHIC SURGERY MAY BE REQUIRED

There are three factors that usually indicate whether an orthodontic or orthopedic case is too extreme to be treated with appliances alone and may require the help of surgery:

- A positive overbite of greater than 8 mm

- A negative overjet (underbite) of greater than 4 mm

- A maxillary transverse discrepancy (crossbite of the upper jaw) greater than 3 mm

Even beyond these guidelines, sometimes a case can still be treated with orthodontics alone. However, if the teeth need to be moved more than 5 mm, then orthognathic surgery typically will be needed to help correct the jaw.

PLANNING ORTHOGNATHIC (CORRECTIVE JAW) SURGERY

When planning treatment, the orthodontist and oral surgeon on the case will meet at least twice before the surgery date to review the case and develop the best plan for bringing the patient's bite as close to ideal as possible. As part of this planning, both doctors follow the FRESH acronym to help them accomplish the major goals of treatment: **F**unction, **R**eliable/realistic, **E**conomic/aesthetic, **S**tability/satisfaction, **H**ealth.

- **Function**: The surgeon and orthodontist should aim for finishing a patient's case with as close to an ideal bite as possible.

- **Reliable**: The surgeon and orthodontist want to use methods of treatment that have been scientifically verified to be highly successful in achieving the correction of skeletal imbalances and that are lower risk. For instance, using rigid fixation to set the jaws after surgery—that is, fixing the bones together using small, permanent titanium plates—instead of just wiring the jaws together.

- **Realistic**: The planned treatment should achieve realistic goals that meet both the patient's and the doctor's expectations.

- **Economic**: The cost of the proposed treatment is always taken into consideration. If the surgery is very expensive, the patient should be aware of this and confirm that he or she can budget for it. Additionally, it should be confirmed that the patient's medical insurance will approve the procedure.

A WORD ON DENTAL INSURANCE AND ORTHOGNATHIC SURGERY

While some dental insurance will cover some of the costs of orthodontic treatment, no dental insurance will cover orthognathic surgery costs—this type of surgery will only be covered by medical insurance.

However, medical insurance can also be difficult, in that insurers will often only cover the orthognathic surgery if the jaw discrepancy is creating a life-threatening situation, which is rarely the case. While large jaw discrepancies may create a functional and aesthetic problem and a poor bite for the patient, very few of these problems will create a life-threatening situation. For these non-life-threatening cases, the choice for surgery is an elective one.

That said, some medical insurance companies *do* cover elective orthognathic surgery, so it's important for the patient and the doctors to find out the amount of coverage for the surgery, if any, before the treatment planning is complete, and definitely before the patient is put into any orthodontic appliances. This is due to the fact that, in many cases, orthodontic appliances are placed before surgery to prepare the teeth for the surgical procedure. During this time, the teeth may look worse and may be less sturdy (decompensated) until the surgical procedure repositions them.

The reason for this is that the teeth will naturally compensate for a bad bite by moving toward each other in an attempt to improve the existing bite. However, as the orthodontist works to put those teeth back in their proper positions prior to surgery—a process that may take six to eighteen months—the actual extent of the skeletal discrepancy between the jaws becomes more evident. During this time, the teeth may look worse until the surgical procedure repositions them.

- **Aesthetic**: The surgery should achieve a dental and facial aesthetic appearance that is pleasing to both the doctor and the patient. In addition, the facial balance should be pleasing both when it's static (sitting still) and when it's dynamic (such as while smiling or talking).

- **Stability**: The surgery should keep the jaw and teeth in positions that are reasonably stable and in balance with the soft tissues. Rigid fixation can help achieve this, such as using small, permanent titanium plates to hold the bone in place, but the surgeon also has to be careful to ensure that the jaws are placed appropriately in the soft tissue envelope.

- **Satisfaction**: Both the orthodontic procedure and the orthognathic surgery should provide the patient and the doctors with a satisfying result that addresses the problems and goals of the treatment. If there were any limitations or downsides to the treatment, the patient should have been made aware of those possibilities before undergoing treatment and satisfied with the information.

- **Health:** Orthodontic and orthognathic surgeries should create a healthier situation in the function and aesthetics of the jaw and facial area, as well as a more comfortable and functional bite for the patient overall.

Planning treatment for a surgical case requires extensive communication and cooperation between the orthodontist and surgeon. Once a proper diagnosis is made, and the FRESH goals and desired outcomes have been established, the next part of the process includes taking a full set of records (photos, x-rays, study models, etc.) and determining exactly where the problem lies in the jaw or jaws in order to make the ideal correction.

PINPOINTING THE PROBLEM

Cephalograms (head x-rays) are the most often patient record studied by orthodontists and orthognathic surgeons, as these images are crucial in indicating where the problem lies in the jaws and what orthodontic treatment should be used to correct it.

When studying cephalograms, the orthodontist and surgeon may find the jaw discrepancy is created more by the lower jaw than the upper. In this case, it would be up to both doctors to determine whether or not only the lower jaw should be moved. If the discrepancy is completely with the lower jaw, the surgeon will indicate only a single jaw surgery is needed. However, even if the discrepancy is only in the lower jaw, it may be so great that the jaw cannot be moved far enough to correct it, in which case both jaws may need to be corrected to bring the mouth into an ideal bite.

For instance, if the upper jaw is set back too far and needs to be advanced, there's only so far it can be moved forward before the nose and lips won't allow further progression, and jaw begins to negatively affect the patient's appearance. In such a case, doctors may recommend surgery on both jaws, moving one jaw partway forward and the other jaw partway back, creating an ideal and balanced result that's both stable and aesthetic.

WHICH SURGERY IS BEST?

There are several different types of corrective jaw surgery and dozens of corrections that may be achieved, from advancements of the upper jaw to downgrafting of the lower jaw, and so on. Additionally, some patients may require more than one type of surgery—or more than one surgical session—to correct their condition. The most common types of orthognathic surgery include the following:

- surgically assisted rapid palatal expansion (SARPE)

- mandibular advancement

- mandibular setback

- maxillary advancement

- maxillary impaction

- maxillomandibular advancement

To determine which surgery is best for the patient, an orthodontist and surgeon will evaluate a patient's soft tissue profile and skeletal structure using a lateral skull x-ray and possibly a 3D cone beam scan, which can show in three dimensions exactly how much each jaw is out of place. They will also perform an in-person exam to determine which of the jaws is the source of the problem.

For the majority of patients, the problem is usually in one jaw or the other, where one is either too large or too small or has grown asymmetrically. In some cases, however, the issue may lay in both jaws, at which point the orthodontist and surgeon will need to decide whether or not both jaws should be treated. For instance, if 80 percent of the discrepancy is in one jaw and 20 percent is in the other, the surgeon may opt to treat only the jaw with the largest discrepancy. This would be especially true if the smaller discrepancy was only a matter of a few millimeters.

Because jaw surgery usually involves larger-scale adjustments of the jaw, it's difficult for orthognathic surgeons to successfully perform micro-adjustments of only a few millimeters. Instead, they would likely overcompensate the one jaw they're working on, moving it more to make up the difference. For example, instead of doing a double jaw surgery and moving one jaw back 2 mm and the other forward 7 mm, the surgeon would simply perform a single jaw surgery and move the latter jaw forward 9 mm to correct the entire discrepancy.

Surgical Approaches

Ultimately, the end goal of both the orthodontist and oral surgeon is to establish a bite that is not only seated properly, but is also aesthetically pleasing. To achieve this, the treatment plan will likely involve one of three common surgical approaches: Le Fort I osteotomy, bilateral sagittal split osteotomy (BSSO), or sliding genioplasty.

LE FORT I OSTEOTOMY

If the discrepancy lies in the mid-face area, such as with an underdeveloped upper jaw, the upper jaw will likely be moved forward using a Le Fort I osteotomy.

Named after Rene Le Fort, who discovered three lines of weaknesses in the facial skeleton in 1901, a Le Fort I osteotomy observes the first line of weakness and separates the bony area located just above the roots of the upper teeth. The operation moves this area either forward or backward depending on the discrepancy, placing the upper jaw in a more ideal position. The jaw is then fixed in place using permanent titanium plates screwed into the bone.

BILATERAL SAGITTAL SPLIT OSTEOTOMY (BSSO)

If the discrepancy is with the lower jaw, such as with a recessed lower jaw or a lower jaw that juts out to far, the surgeon and orthodontist might opt for a BSSO. This approach involves cutting the lower jaw diagonally, about half an inch behind the last molar, and sliding it in the appropriate direction—either backward or forward. Once the jaw is in the correct position, it's fixed in place using permanent titanium plates and screws.

SLIDING GENIOPLASTY

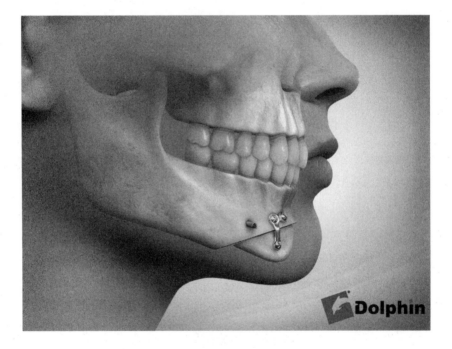

Chin deformities also exist in the lower face, independent of the size of the lower jaw. In these cases, the chin bone can be sectioned away from the lower jaw and slid either forward or backward as needed and permanently fixed into place with titanium plates and screws.

"BRACING" FOR PRE- AND POST-SURGERY

Before undergoing any surgery, patients first need to go through a round of wearing braces or Invisalign to position (decompensate) their teeth in a way that allows the surgeon to move the jaw or jaws into the best possible position. This process can take anywhere from six to eighteen months before the surgery, depending on the discrepancy. While this may seem like a long time, the more the teeth are prepared for surgery, the more likely it is the surgeon will do a more accurate job, which can help reduce the amount of time spent on post-surgical orthodontics.

After the surgery, patients will likely need to wear braces or Invisalign for an additional six to eighteen months, until their jaw and bite are in the best possible position and the healing process is complete. If the patient is wearing Invisalign, he or she will also have surgical arch bars placed on the teeth, which will allow the surgeon to hold the teeth together using elastics or rubber bands during the healing process.

Specific Orthognathic Surgeries

SURGICALLY ASSISTED RAPID PALATAL EXPANSION (SARPE)

SARPE is one of the more common procedures used to correct narrow upper jaws and posterior crossbites. This procedure is usually performed once a patient is fully grown and the upper jaw has fused at the sutures, making it difficult or impossible to expand the jaw without surgery.

Once diagnosed and a treatment plan has been made, a rapid palatal expander (RPE) device is custom-made to fit the patient's teeth and is cemented onto the upper molars. The patient then undergoes a Le Fort I osteotomy to "release" the upper jaw into two halves. Immediately after surgery, a small screw in the RPE is turned, and the patient is instructed to turn the screw twice a day—a process that expands the palate by about half a millimeter each day until the desired width is achieved.

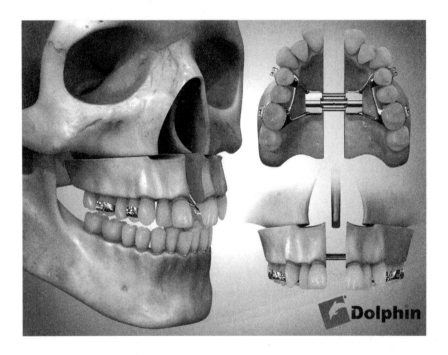

Once the upper jaw is the correct width, the RPE is left in place for six to seven months while the bone heals and new bone fills in the gaps. Afterward, the RPE is removed, and the patient remains in braces until the bite is as close as possible to ideal.

MAXILLARY ADVANCEMENT
OR SETBACK SURGERY

Maxillary Advancements or setback surgeries are commonly used to correct overjets (buck teeth), anterior crossbites (underbite), and midline discrepancies.

Class 3 discrepancies—more commonly known as significant underbites—are present in about 0.6 percent of the US population, or around 1.9 million people. Of these, about a third are severe enough to warrant surgery.

In these cases, a Le Fort I osteotomy is conducted to move the upper jaw either backward or forward, depending on the discrepancy; the upper jaw is then fixed in a more normal position.

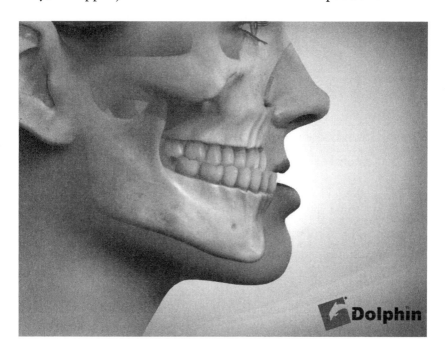

MAXILLARY IMPACTION (OR DOWNGRAFTING) SURGERY

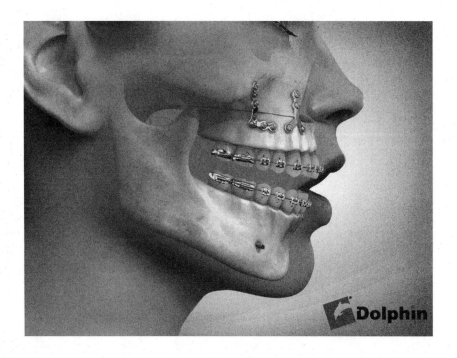

Downgrafting surgery is commonly used to correct vertical excesses (gummy smiles) or vertical deficiencies ("overclosed" or hidden upper teeth). The condition of having a long, narrow upper face is often due to an upper jaw that grew too long vertically. Patients with this condition also tend to have very gummy smiles, with 5–6 mm of gum tissue showing when they smile, although there have been cases of patients showing in excess of 20 mm of gum line when smiling, resulting in smiles that show more gum than tooth.

Conversely, other patients may present with an "overclosed" upper face, where the upper jaw hasn't grown downward enough and the front teeth disappear under the upper lip.

In either case, a modified Le Fort I osteotomy can be done to either reduce (impact) the vertical height of the upper jaw to reduce a gummy smile or to add bone—typically taken from the patient's hip—to increase the height of the upper jaw (downgraft) so that the patient's upper teeth become visible.

MANDIBULAR ADVANCEMENT (OR SETBACK) SURGERY

Of the two mandibular, or lower jaw, surgeries, mandibular advancement is far more common, especially as our awareness of the condition of sleep apnea—a sleep disorder characterized by sudden and frequent stops in breathing—grows. If the lower jaw is set too far back in the mouth, for instance, it may constrict the airway and cause sleep apnea to become worse.

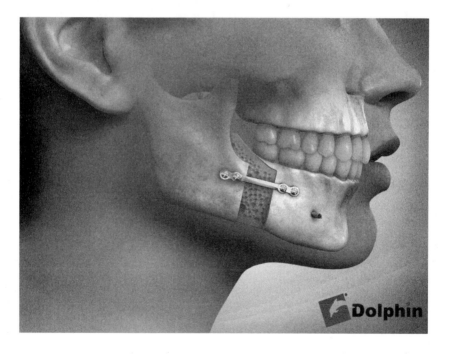

Class 2 lower jaw deficiencies, such as recessed or protruding lower jaws, occur in about 10 percent of the US population, and of those, only about 5 percent are severe enough to warrant surgery. The majority of these conditions require mandibular advancement surgery rather than mandibular setback surgery.

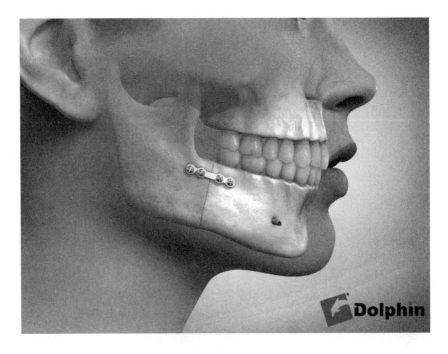

To correct a recessed or protruding lower jaw, a BSSO (Bilateral Sagittal Split Osteotomy) can be done to slide the lower jaw either backward or forward, depending on the discrepancy.

MAXILLOMANDIBULAR ADVANCEMENT

This procedure is a double jaw advancement surgery designed to open up the airway to the maximum volume possible to help correct sleep apnea. In these cases, the upper jaw is not only moved forward using a Le Fort I osteotomy but is often set slightly further down toward the back of the upper jaw. The lower jaw is also moved forward using a BSSO and adjusted so that the chin rotates upward and connects properly with the newly adjusted upper jaw.

This surgery increases the airway volume not only in the nasal pharynx area but also in the lower oral pharynx area, which is why it is one of the main surgeries for patients suffering from sleep apnea.

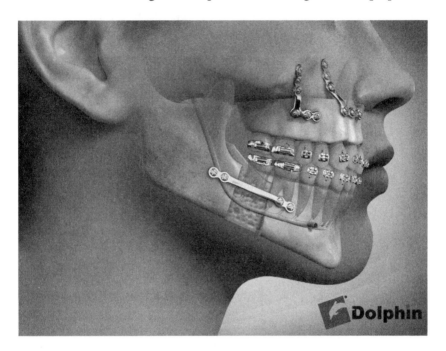

RECOVERY FROM ORTHOGNATHIC SURGERY

After any given corrective jaw surgery, recovery time for the soft tissues can take anywhere from two to four weeks for the swelling to go down and the flesh to heal. The jaws mend slower, often taking between three and four months for the bones to completely heal.

Immediately following jaw surgery, a patient will often have interarch elastics placed to help keep the bite together. In the past, patients typically had their jaws wired shut—a practice which finally ended in the 1990s, as it proved to be very dangerous for the patient.

For instance, if the patient became nauseous following surgery, the inability to open the mouth could create a life-threatening situation.

Additionally, recent studies have found that patients who can conservatively move their jaws after surgery are able to heal quicker. Because of this, some surgeons will fit jaw surgery patients with removable rubber bands that hold the jaw in place until the patient removes them in order to eat or speak. Other surgeons will fit a recovering jaw surgery patient with a splint (a tray that appears similar to a mouth guard) that the patient wears for the first two to three weeks to help establish stability. These splints can either be custom designed using CAD/CAM technology or be created from acrylic, using study models.

While rigid fixation, such as small titanium plates, has been used to help increase the stability of the jaw while healing, the jaw can still move slightly, so it is important to use whatever stabilizing device is recommended by the surgeon to help keep the jaws and teeth together during those important first few weeks.

BREAKDOWN OF SURGICAL RECOVERY

Seven days post-surgery: The patient will be on interarch elastics, with or without a splint, depending on the case. They can usually do some voluntary opening of the mouth by removing the elastics.

Two weeks post-surgery: The patient can perform passive exercises, such as opening as wide as they can without pain and doing gentle movements of the jaw by moving it up and down and back and forth.

Two to four weeks post-surgery: If the patient still has pain, the surgeon may indicate additional therapies, such as muscle massage, a home exercise program, physical therapy, ultrasound, and the application of heat and ice to the area.

Eight weeks post-surgery: The patient will typically undergo the finishing movements of the orthodontic treatment, and their functioning will return to normal. If not already placed, braces with rubber bands may be added to bring the bite into its ideal position.

Four months post-surgery: The jawbones have typically healed by this point, and the braces can likely come off.

Chapter 7 Summary

- Accelerated orthodontic procedures make it possible for tooth movement to occur 50–75 percent faster than normal.

- Treatment time with accelerated orthodontics can be affected by the complexity of the case, the amount of tooth movement required, the amount of patient cooperation required, and the patient's biological response to the procedure.

- The most effective accelerated orthodontic procedures are decortication micro-osteoperforation.

- Decortication, or removing part of the alveolar bone and replacing it with a bone graft, can cause the teeth to move 50–75 percent faster than normal during the bone's two-month healing phase.

- Micro-osteoperforation—the process of drilling a series of very fine holes into the alveolar bone—can cause the teeth near the perforations to move at an increased rate of 50–75 percent during the healing period, which lasts between eight and sixteen weeks.

- Low-level mechanical vibrations from using a vibrational pulsating device, such as Acceledent, does not have enough research to show that it actually accelerates treatment. Most studies show that it does not.

- Faster tooth movement decreases many of the risks associated with orthodontic treatment, such as susceptibility to cavities, increased root resorption, gingivitis, periodontitis, and other gum and bone diseases.

- If a significant jaw discrepancy isn't caught early enough (typically during the first fourteen to eighteen years of a person's life), then surgery may be the only option.

- The three conditions that usually require orthognathic (corrective jaw) surgery are a positive overjet greater than 8 mm, a negative overjet of greater than 4 mm, or a crossbite of the upper jaw greater than 3 mm.

- Jaw surgery usually involves larger-scale adjustments of the jaw. The most common types of orthognathic surgery are the following:

  □ surgically assisted rapid palatal expansion (SARPE)

- □ mandibular advancement

- □ mandibular setback

- □ maxillary advancement

- □ maxillary impaction

- □ maxillomandibular advancement

- Surgical patients often need to wear braces for anywhere from six to eighteen months both before and after surgery.

- Using an oral appliance to manage sleep apnea should be used in conjunction with a tooth positioner to help minimize unwanted tooth movement.

Sleep Apnea

A person can go three weeks without food and three days without water, but no more than three minutes without air. The path air takes to get into our lungs—through the nasal airway, trachea, throat, and especially, the mouth—is where orthodontists spend most of their time observing. Because of their specialization with these areas, it gives them a strategic position to intervene when airway complications are either identified or start to develop, such as with the sleeping disorder obstructive sleep apnea (OSA).

Now more than ever, sleep apnea awareness is an important aspect of orthodontics, as the profession plays a larger role in diagnosing and treating airway obstructions. This is because orthodontists, who typically see patients for the first time at age seven, are in a key place to identify an abnormal growth of the jaws or craniofacial complex (the area comprising the head, face, and oral cavity).

During an exam, an orthodontist will usually take x-rays of the head that include the entire upper airway, from the nose to the trachea. If there are any obstructions, the orthodontist will be able to spot them. Additionally, more orthodontists are incorporating 3D cone beam technology into their exams, which gives them a deeper look into how patients' upper airways are developing, as well as the ability to measure important factors, such as the patient's minimum airway volume. This allows the orthodontist to pinpoint where the airway constriction is occurring.

WHAT CAUSES OSA?

In 1872, C.V. Tomes was the first to describe how obstructed breathing could influence the shape of the face, coining the term "adenoid facies" to describe the long, open-mouthed face of children whose enlarged adenoids caused an upper airway obstruction, forcing them to breathe through their mouths. Since then, orthodontists have been looking for both structural and functional factors in the jaws, head, face, oral cavity, and upper airway that could influence that area's growth, form, and function.

In 1962, the study of this subject led anatomy professor Melvin Moss to develop his *functional matrix hypothesis*, which states that bones are grown based on function instead of form; they grow to fulfill prior needs instead of growing a certain way simply because they're genetically programmed to do so. This hypothesis led Moss to theorize that nasal breathing allowed for the proper growth of the head, face, and oral cavity. If that nasal breathing is inhibited, then this area—the head, face, and oral cavity—will not fully develop.

For instance, if young patients are forced to constantly breathe through their mouths because their nasal airways are blocked, then they are likely to develop a narrow upper jaw and relaxed muscle tone, because the tongue does not have the opportunity to sit as it normally would against the palate, where it would help to shape the width of the upper jaw.

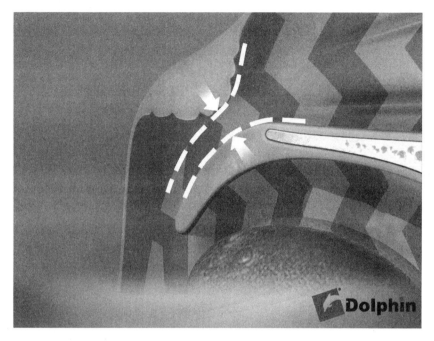

In some cases, the adenoid tissue becomes enlarged and constricts the airway with the soft palate.

As a result, patients develop a narrow palate and a posterior crossbite, and their lower jaw will likely develop more "downward" than it should, creating a large overjet of the teeth. Moreover, the patient will also likely develop a narrow base of the nose, proclined upper incisors (front teeth that stick out), a proclined lower lip (a lower lip that juts out), a high palate, and aretrognathic mandible (a recessed lower jaw/chin). These issues tend to promote a vacant facial expression.

This condition can be improved almost immediately in young patients by removing the obstruction and returning nasal breathing to normal. However, if the obstruction isn't removed until a patient is older and is done growing (in the late teens or early twenties), then there may be little to no change after the obstruction is removed, and surgery may be required to correct the skeletal discrepancies between the jaws.

Apart from enlarged adenoids, OSA can also be caused by unusual upper airway blockages such as the following:

- nasal septum deviations

- turbinate hypertrophy (enlargement of the bony structures on the side walls of the inside of the nose)

- nasal polyps

- mid-face hypoplasia (underdevelopment of the upper jaw, cheek bones, and eye sockets that can result in a severe underbite)

- fetal hypoplasia

- macroglossia (enlarged tongue)

- retrognathia (recessed chin/lower jaw)

- micrognathia (undersized lower jaw)

- tumors that may be blocking or causing a narrowing of the airway

IS SNORING A SIGN OF SLEEP APNEA?

About 7 percent of men and 3 percent of women have OSA.[24] While most patients with OSA will show signs of snoring, not everyone who snores has OSA. In fact, snoring is usually caused by the split-second closure of the upper airway, it doesn't cause the snorer to stop breathing. Snorers with OSA, however, may stop breathing for significant lengths of time (also called *apneas*), leading to sleep fragmentation, hypoxemia (low oxygen in the blood), or both. Other signs and symptoms of OSA include the following:

- excessive sleepiness
- fatigue
- memory impairment
- mood disturbance
- decreased libido
- social withdrawal
- cardiovascular disease
- lower jaw is too small or is set too far back
- presence of hypertension
- BMI of thirty or higher
- neck circumference of seventeen inches or larger
- observed choking or gasping during sleep

---

24 Naresh M. Punjabi, "The Epidemiology of Adult Obstructive Sleep Apnea," *Proceedings of the American Thoracic Society* 5, no. 2 (2008): 136–143.

- inattention and changes in energy levels during the day

- enlarged tonsils and/or adenoids

There is also growing evidence that patients who clench and grind their teeth or have abnormal tongue positions during sleep may also have some degree of OSA.[25] These parafunctional activities may be related to patients' attempts to keep their airway open during sleep, moving their jaw around or clenching their teeth in order to keep the muscles in the neck and throat activated and their airway open. Additionally, moving the tongue into an abnormal position, such as between the teeth or pushing against the teeth, can also help to keep the airway open.

If patients show any of these signs or symptoms, ortho-dontists will often advise that they undergo screening tests to determine whether they should see a sleep specialist for a sleep study, also called a polysomnog-raphy (PSG).

DIAGNOSING OSA

The only way to properly diagnose someone with OSA is to perform a sleep study, or PSG; however, PSGs typically have to receive approval

---

25   Oksenberg, A. and Arons, E., "Sleep bruxism related to obstructive sleep apnea: the effect of continuous positive airway pressure," *Sleep Med* 3, no. 6 (2002): 513-5; Macaluso, G.M., Guerra, et al., "Sleep bruxism is a disorders related to periodic arousals during sleep," *J Dent Res.* 77 (1998): 565–573; Kato, T., et al., "Sleep bruxism: an oromotor activity secondary to micro-arousal," *J Dent Res.* 80 (2001):1940–1944.

from medical insurance before being conducted, which means the procedure must first be recommended by a doctor. Before making a PSG recommendation, the doctor will likely perform one or more of these basic screening tests:

- **Epworth Sleepiness Questionnaire:** This tool presents patients with eight situations, determining their likelihood of falling asleep in each. These situations are scored on a scale of zero to three, with the total score being twenty-four.

- **Cephalometric Analysis:** An x-ray of the skull used to evaluate dental and skeletal relationships, as well as the relationship between bony and soft tissue landmarks, in order to identify any growth abnormalities.

- **Cone Beam CT Analysis**: A 3D x-ray that measures minimum airway volume (MAV).

- **STOP-BANG Questionnaire:** An acronym for "snoring, tired, observed pressure, body mass index, age, neck circumference, and gender," this questionnaire is a basic assessment of sleep habits and physical factors that could contribute to OSA.

- **Berlin Questionnaire:** This tool is ten questions designed to predict the severity of a patient's OSA.

- **Intraoral Evaluation**: A standard oral exam, which can include an evaluation of the airway and any potential visible obstructions.

- **Take-Home Sleep Monitor:** These monitors, such as the NOX-T3, will measure key parameters like blood oxygen saturation, apnea and hypopnea episodes, and disturbed breathing patterns. While it's not a definitive test for OSA, it is one of the more efficient prescreening tests for this condition.

All of these questionnaires and analyses are meant to help the clinician screen patients and assess their risk level for OSA before recommending a PSG. If the results do point to a potential OSA diagnosis, the patient will be scheduled for a PSG, which involves an overnight sleep study at sleep center under the supervision of a qualified technician and sleep expert, who will use a variety of monitors to measure the patient's sleep quality.

While a PSG measures dozens of factors during sleep, the main measurement for determining OSA is the patient's apnea-hypopnea index (AHI). This measurement provides the clinician with exactly how many apneas (breathing cessation) and hypopneas (abnormally shallow breathing) the patient is experience each hour during sleep.

Another important factor a PSG measures is the patient's respiratory disturbance index (RDI), which is the total number of events (apneas, hypopneas, and RERAs, or respiratory effort related arousals) that a patient experiences each hour. The RDI measurement is generally higher than the AHI because it includes the frequency of RERAs, while the AHI does not.

WHAT DOES A POLYSOMNOGRAPH (PSG) MEASURE?

A PSG takes dozens of measurements while a patient is sleeping, from eye movement to heartbeat to breathing. Among the many parameters monitored are the following:

- oxygen saturation

- brain waves

- muscle movement

- eye movement/rapid eye movement

- airflow (both oral and nasal)

- temperature

- heart rate

- pulse

- breathing efforts (both in the throat and abdomen)

- CO_2 levels of the skin

- snoring

- limb movements

- air pressure in the esophagus

UPPER AIRWAY RESISTANCE SYNDROME

Patients with RERAs tend to have frequent micro-arousals of three seconds or less during sleep, and too many RERAs per night are associated with daytime sleepiness. Some patients may have RERAs but not apneas or hypopneas, which likely means that the patient is experiencing some increased resistance in the airway but that it's not necessarily closing all the way, as it would with OSA. This condition, called *upper airway resistance syndrome,* is a milder form of OSA and can also be identified with a PSG.

ORTHODONTIC TREATMENT FOR OSA

Once OSA has been diagnosed with a PSG, there are a number of orthodontic treatments, both surgical and nonsurgical, that may help open the upper airway temporarily and/or permanently.

LIFESTYLE AND BEHAVIOR MODIFICATION

While not a primary means of treatment, lifestyle and behavior modifications can help reduce the severity of OSA. These modifications can include the following:

- weight loss—exercises that can lead to a healthier BMI of twenty-five or less

- positional therapy—using props or behavioral therapy to avoid sleeping on the back, which can increase the severity of OSA

- avoiding alcohol or sedatives before going to bed

CPAP MACHINE

Standing for *continuous positive airway pressure*, the CPAP device consists of a nose or mouth piece (or nose and mouth piece) through which compressed air is blown. This positive flow of air holds the airway open by not allowing the soft tissues to collapse during sleep.

While the CPAP is the most prescribed therapy for OSA and is considered the gold standard for OSA treatment, it's also the least tolerated therapy. Many patients find it uncomfortable to wear and even more uncomfortable to fall asleep while wearing. This may be due to wearing the mask all night, the pressure on the airway, or irritation to the nasal and upper airway tissues, but in any case, the machine can make it difficult to fall asleep.

ORAL APPLIANCE THERAPY

Oral appliances are considered a very viable option for patients who cannot tolerate CPAP therapy. There are several types of appliances out there, and all are designed to hold the lower jaw in a forward position. In doing so, the tongue, which is attached to the lower jaw, is also held forward, creating a larger space between the base of the tongue and the back of the throat, increasing the upper airway volume exactly where most patients have a constriction. These devices are also easier to use and are much more portable than CPAP machines.

TYPES OF ORAL APPLIANCES

- **Tongue Retention Device**: Designed to treat mild OSA, this device holds the tongue in a forward position in the mouth, typically between the teeth.

- **Soft-Palate Lifting Device**: Also for treating milder forms of OSA, this device is designed to hold the soft palate up and prevent it from collapsing during sleep.

- **Mandibular Advancement Splints**: For moderate to severe OSA, these devices—including the MARA, Herbst, and Twin Block appliances (see Chapter 5 for more on these devices)—hold the lower jaw and tongue forward, helping the airway remain open during sleep. The effectiveness of these splints can be tested with a PSG, or the patient can wear the appliance during a cone beam CT scan to assess how much it's affecting airway volume. However, because these appliances rely on the teeth for retention, they are not recommended for use by patients with periodontal issues, as the appliance could harm the integrity of the teeth. Additionally, patients with TMJ issues should not use these appliances, as they may exacerbate the condition. Patients with severe gag reflexes and poor manual dexterity should also avoid using these devices. There are also several side effects from the long-term use of mandibular advancement splints:

□ dry mouth

□ excessive salivation

□ tooth discomfort

□ gingival irritation

□ jaw muscle tenderness

□ TMJ discomfort

□ changes in bite due to teeth shifting from the pressure placed on them by the appliance*

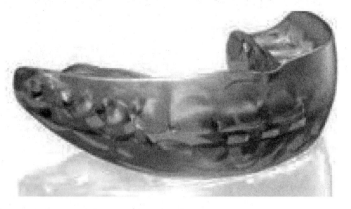

*This last side effect can often be managed by wearing a **tooth positioner**—a device that resembles a large sports mouth guard—for twenty to thirty minutes per day to keep the patients' teeth in their original position. The positioner acts as a retainer to help correct any movement of the teeth that may occur while using oral appliance therapy (OAT).

While oral appliances were not prescribed to patients with severe OSA in the past, these devices have improved tremendously over the years, and clinicians are finding that today's oral appliances are producing positive results similar to those achieved with CPAP therapy, even in patients with severe OSA. Today, approximately 40 percent of patients with OSA are successfully treated with oral appliance therapy, with at least another 25 percent showing a partial reduction in OSA, resulting in at least two-thirds of patients experiencing some degree of OSA improvement with oral appliance therapy.

UPPER AIRWAY ELECTRICAL STIMULATION (UAES)

This implantable device is more of a long-term fix for OSA that delivers a mild stimulation to the nerve that controls the tongue (the hypoglossal nerve) to keep the airway open. The UAES is implanted in the chest, much like a pacemaker, and can be turned on before bed with a remote control. When activated, the device automatically senses if the patient stops breathing and stimulates the tongue to move. In most clinical trials, this device has shown a 68 percent decrease in patients' AHI scores. While this treatment is mainly reserved for those who can't tolerate CPAP machines or oral appliance therapy, it's also not recommended for patients with an AHI above sixty-five and/or a BMI above sixty-two.

MAXILLOMANDIBULAR (DOUBLE-JAW) ADVANCEMENT SURGERY

Over the past few years, combined advancement of the upper and lower jaws have become the surgical treatment gold standard for treatment of OSA in patients with decreased oral-pharyngeal airways, whom studies have shown are more likely to suffer from pharyngeal collapse. By surgically moving both the upper and lower jaws forward, the airway is opened up, and the muscles and tendons are tightened, reducing the risk of collapse.

This surgery has the added benefit of not only correcting abnormal measurements that lead to OSA, such as an airway space of less than 11 mm and a hyoid bone angle of greater than fifteen degrees, but also helping correct any facial or bite deformities that the patient may be suffering from.

TONSILLECTOMY AND ADENOIDECTOMY

These surgeries, when done at a younger age, have shown to be highly effective in treating pediatric OSA, resolving an average of 82 percent of cases.

LESS COMMON OSA TREATMENTS

TRACHEOSTOMY

This procedure creates a small opening in the trachea below the obstruction so that the patient can breathe. This is mainly done in extreme cases of OSA and/or for patients who are not good candidates for the CPAP, oral appliance therapy, or double jaw surgery.

NASAL PROCEDURES

If the obstruction causing the OSA is mainly in the nasal area, procedures such as septoplasty (correction of the cartilage that divides the two sides of the nose), functional rhinoplasty (correction of the nose), nasal turbinate reduction, and nasal polyp removal can be used to open up the nasal airway.

UVULOPALATOPHARYNGOPLASTY

This procedure involves the surgical removal of a portion of the soft palate in the uvula (the fleshy tissue that hangs down in the back of your mouth), helping open up the upper pharyngeal airway. While this procedure is useful in reducing snoring, it's typically not as effective as other therapies and surgeries for reducing OSA.

RADIO FREQUENCY ABLATION

This technique causes a hardening of the soft palate and uvula, a process that can help prevent the soft tissues from collapsing during sleep.

COULD A TOOTH EXTRACTION MAKE OSA WORSE?

There is a growing concern that the removal of a tooth or teeth that results in the front teeth moving back can result in less space for the tongue, which in turn could move the tongue further back in the mouth and constrict the airway, contributing to the risk for OSA. However, even in cases where the tooth extractions are closed by retracting the front teeth, there's often very little—if any—change in airway volume.

For instance, in a study[26] of sixty-two patients, half of whom had their first four bicuspids removed for orthodontic treatment, there was no significant difference in airway volume between those patients who had their teeth extracted and those who had not. Another study, conducted by Valiathan et al.,[27] showed that there is no significant change to the minimum airway volume after first bicuspids are removed and the site is closed by moving the front teeth back.

THE IMPORTANCE OF A MULTIDISCIPLINARY APPROACH TO TREATING OSA

Several types of doctors are key in the process of screening and testing for OSA. During this screening process, it's important not only to ask the right questions and properly identify the various signs and symptoms, but also to involve the right doctors.

---

26   N Stefanovic et al., "Three-dimensional pharyngeal airway changes in orthodontic patients treated with and without extractions," *Orthod Craniofacial Res* 16, no. 2 (2013): 87–96, doi:10.1111/ocr.12009.

27   M Valiathan et al., "Effects of extraction versus non-extraction treatment on oropharyngeal airway volume," *Angle Orthod*, (2010): 1068–74.

PEDIATRICIAN

From the time children are born, they see a pediatrician, who is in an ideal place for recognizing the signs and symptoms of OSA at a very young age. Symptoms can include sleepiness during the day, feeling tired or fatigued early in the day, the inability to play sports due to lack of energy, and even ADHD, with the lack of sleep contributing to the child's inability to focus or concentrate.

If a pediatrician is concerned about the possibility of OSA in a patient, he or she can perform a Mallampati test, which classifies the soft tissue in the palate on a scale of one to four. One is ideal, with a large opening between the soft palate, tongue, and tonsillar pillars, while four means that the edges of the soft palate and the opening to the throat are either not very visible or are not visible at all, which would indicate an airway issue.

While the Mallampati test was originally developed to determine the ease of placing a breathing tube in a patient's throat, on average, for every point increase in the Mallampati score, the risk of OSA increased by more than twofold, and the AHI increased by more than five events per hour.

THE MALLAMPATI SCORE

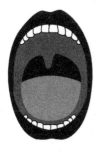 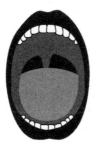 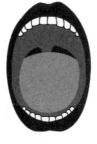 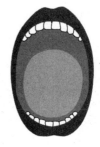

CLASS I
Complete visualization
of the soft palate

CLASS II
Complete visualization
of the uvula

CLASS III
Visualization of only
the base of the uvula

CLASS VI
Soft palate is not
visible at all

PEDIATRIC DENTIST

Pediatric dentists will often see children as early as one year old and can identify several signs and symptoms of OSA starting at this age:

- excessive grinding and clenching of teeth

- excessive wear on the teeth

- teeth that are cracked, fractured, or chipped from clenching

- parafunctional tongue habits, such as pushing on the teeth

ORTHODONTIST

Children should typically start seeing an orthodontist by age seven. The orthodontist will usually perform a lateral cephalogram (skull x-ray) and analysis to measure the patient's airway, as well as the patient's hard tissue development and skeletal patterns.

ENT (EAR, NOSE, AND THROAT) DOCTOR

While some young children may not see an ENT unless recommended by their pediatrician, it's a good idea to have them evaluated by an ENT if they are presenting any of the symptoms of OSA. The ENT would be able to do a more in-depth evaluation of the upper airway, specifically checking the nasal passages, adenoids, and tonsils for any issues.

When it comes to properly diagnosing and treating OSA, teamwork is essential, from an orthodontic screening, to physician referral for diagnosing and monitoring during orthodontic treatment, to airway outcomes and beyond. The involvement of and coordination between these different specialists will create specific responsibilities for testing and monitoring and will provide a much more well-rounded approach to treatment.

Above all, it's important to address all of the patient's needs, checking on their overall health, their specific dental health, and the various factors that can play a role in OSA, including the skeletal structure, the patient's bite, airway volume, nasal passages, and the condition of the adenoids, tonsils, and throat.

Chapter 8 Summary

- Orthodontists are strategically positioned to intervene with airway complications, such as obstructive sleep apnea (OSA).

- OSA can be caused by enlarged adenoids; excessive mouth-breathing in young children, causing a narrow jaw to develop; or unusual upper airway blockages.

- About 7 percent of men and 3 percent of women have OSA.

- With OSA, a person may stop breathing during sleep for significant lengths of time (called *apneas*), leading to sleep fragmentation, low blood oxygen levels, or both.

- OSA is most commonly diagnosed with a sleep study using a polysomnography (PSG). Before recommending a PSG, a doctor will likely perform a screening test, such as the Epworth Sleepiness Questionnaire or an intraoral evaluation.

- A PSG measures dozens of factors while patients are sleeping, from their pulse to the air pressure in their esophagus. It also gauges their respiratory disturbance index (RDI).

- Common OSA treatment options include lifestyle and behavior modification, CPAP machines, oral appliance therapy, upper airway electrical stimulation, maxillomandibular (double jaw) advancement surgery, tonsillectomy, and adenoidectomy.

- Despite common belief, tooth extractions have very little, if any, impact on airway volume.

- Several doctors are key in screening and testing for OSA, and it is important to involve the right ones in the process. These doctors include pediatricians, pediatric dentists, orthodontists, and ear, nose, and throat (ENT) doctors.

truly hope you've enjoyed the book, but more importantly, I hope you have a better understanding of orthodontic treatment. Overall, I hope that I've helped to dispel many of the myths and misconceptions that exist around orthodontics.

While there have been many advances in orthodontic treatment over the years, the mouth and teeth have not changed; they still adhere to the same biological principles they always have. If these principles are ignored in favor of some fad treatment that has nothing but anecdotal evidence supporting its effectiveness, the risks that you take during orthodontic treatment increase dramatically.

WHAT TO LOOK FOR IN A GOOD ORTHODONTIST

When looking for your own orthodontist, make sure they have these two important qualifications:

- The orthodontist is board-certified (this means that his or her outcomes and skills have been assessed by some of the most knowledgeable orthodontists in the country)

- He or she has several years of experience and a strong grasp of the latest technology. Even though using the latest technology doesn't always equate with great results, the most current technologies are likely at least help improve the efficiency of the treatment.

GETTING A SECOND OPINION

When consulting with an orthodontist about a procedure, if the recommendation is a two-phase treatment, always ask if it's possible to accomplish the same result in one phase. Two phases are rarely needed and only increase the risk associated with orthodontic treatment, as well as increasing the cost by an additional 25–75 percent.

If a two-phase treatment or surgical orthodontics is recommended, consider getting a second opinion. There may be other options available. Additionally, if one orthodontist tells you that a certain appliance, such as Invisalign, won't work for you, it may be that the practitioner doesn't have the experience to make the appliance work, not that you're a poor candidate. This is also an appropriate question to ask another orthodontist.

INFORMATION AND COMPLIMENTARY CONSULTATIONS

For more information on any of the principles or procedures you've read about in this book, please visit www.drdantegonzales.com. If you're in the Dublin, California, area, call our offices for a complimentary consultation at 925-230-0099.